Praise for
Every Man's Battle and *Every Young Man's Battle*
by Stephen Arterburn, Fred Stoeker, and Mike Yorkey

"There is no more common enemy of true manhood than the diversion or the perversion of our sexual capacities. I welcome every contribution to the arsenal of resistance."

—JACK W. HAYFORD, LITTD, pastor of the Church on the Way
and president of the King's Seminary

"This book will revolutionize the marriage of every man who reads it. Why? Because every man battles sexual temptations and every marriage grows stronger when these temptations are defeated. The vulnerable, honest, and insightful pages of this book reveal what every man must know."

—DRS. LES AND LESLIE PARROTT, authors of *Saving Your
Marriage Before It Starts*

"This timely resource presents clear practical principles for sexual purity. Arterburn and Stoeker call for courage, commitment, and self-discipline as they lead men into a more successful relationship with God, family, and spouse. This book is truly for every man."

—DR. JOHN C. MAXWELL, founder of the INJOY Group

"God has used Steve Arterburn countless times to impact my heart and life; I am thankful for him and his investment in *Every Man's Battle.* I am also grateful for Fred Stoeker. Fred pours himself into this book with honesty, vulnerability, and a practical strategy to fight the good fight. He offers biblical truth and hope to anyone with ears to hear how to battle the war of sexual temptation. Read with an open heart—*Every Man's Battle* may save your marriage and your witness."

—DR. GARY ROSBERG, president of America's Family Coaches
and author of *Guard Your Heart* and *The Five Love Needs of
Men and Women*

Stephen Arterburn
Fred Stoeker with Mike Yorkey

every single man's battle

Staying on the Path of Sexual Purity

A Guide for Personal or Group Study

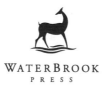

WATERBROOK
PRESS

EVERY SINGLE MAN'S BATTLE
PUBLISHED BY WATERBROOK PRESS
2375 Telstar Drive, Suite 160
Colorado Springs, Colorado 80920
A division of Random House Inc.

Details in some anecdotes and stories have been changed to protect the identities of the persons involved.

ISBN 1-4000-7128-3

Published in association with the literary agency of Alive Communications Inc., 7680 Goddard Street, Suite 200, Colorado Springs, CO 80920.

Printed in the United States of America
2005—First Edition

10 9 8 7 6 5 4 3 2 1

contents

questions you may have
about this workbook

What will *Every Single Man's Battle* workbook do for me?

This workbook will guide you through some serious Bible study, an intense examination of your personal life, and an honest application of biblical truth to help you win the war on sexual temptation and live a pure life in God's way.

You'll find realistic help straight from God's Word for training your eyes and your mind to increasingly see and think according to God's standards.

Is this workbook enough or do I also need the book *Every Man's Battle*?

In the studies you'll find excerpts from the book *Every Man's Battle,* each one marked at the beginning and end by this symbol: 📖. Those excerpts crystallize key points from the chapters in *Every Man's Battle.* But still, to get the most out of this supplementary workbook, you need to read along in the book *Every Man's Battle* every week. You'll find the appropriate chapters to read listed at the beginning of each weekly session.

What's the purpose for the introductory material at the beginning of the book and before every lesson?

The authors recognize that the battle for sexual purity among single men is different in significant ways from the battle faced by married men. As a result specific material has been included to help single men face the tough challenges of maintaining sexual integrity in a sex-soaked culture.

The lessons look long. Do I need to work through everything in each one?

This workbook is designed to promote your thorough exploration of all the content, but you may find it best to focus your time and discussion on some sections and questions more than others. To help your pacing, we've designed the workbook so it can most easily be used in either an eight-week or a twelve-week approach.

- *For the eight-week track,* simply follow the basic organization already set up with the eight different weekly sessions.
- *For the twelve-week track,* the lessons labeled as sessions two, five, six, and seven can be divided into two parts (you'll see the dividing place marked in the text).

In addition, of course, you may decide to follow a different pace—faster or slower—whether you're going through the workbook individually or as part of a group.

Above all, keep in mind that the purpose of this workbook is to help guide you in specific life application of the biblical truths taught in *Every Man's Battle.* The broad questions included in each weekly study are meant to help you approach this practical application from different angles and with personal reflection and self-examination. Allowing adequate time to prayerfully reflect on each question will be much more valuable for you than rushing through the workbook.

How do I bring together a small group to go through this workbook?
You can go through this workbook on your own, if you want, and no doubt it will do you some good. But we have to say—you'll get far more out of this workbook if you're able to go through it with a small group of like-minded single men. As we point out in the opening chapters, connecting with others and connecting with God are the keys to living a life of sexual purity as a single person.

What do you do if you don't know of any group that's going through this workbook? Start such a group on your own! If you take a copy of the book *Every Man's Battle,* plus a copy of this supplementary workbook, and show them to the single Christian men you know, you'll be surprised at how many will indicate interest in joining you for exploring this topic together.

And it doesn't require a long commitment from them. The workbook is clearly set up so you complete one lesson per week and finish in only eight weeks—or, if you'd like to proceed at a little slower pace, you can follow the instructions provided for covering the exact same content in a twelve-week track.

Your once-per-week meeting could happen during the lunch hour one day at work, in the early morning before work begins, on a weekday evening, or even on a Saturday morning. The location could be an office or meeting room at work, a room at a club or restaurant, a classroom at church, or someone's basement or den at home. Choose a location where your discussion won't be overheard by others so the men are comfortable in sharing candidly and freely.

This workbook follows a simple, easy-to-use design. First, each man in the group completes a week's lesson on his own. Then, when you come together that week, you discuss together the group questions provided under the Every Man's Talk heading in each week's lesson. Of course, if you have time, you can also discuss at length any of the other questions or topics in that week's lesson; we guarantee the men in your group will find these to be worth exploring. And they're likely as well to have plenty of their own related questions to bring up for discussion.

It's best if one person in your group is designated as the facilitator. This person is *not* a lecturer or teacher but simply has the responsibility to keep the discussion moving and to ensure that each man in the group has the opportunity to join in fully.

At the beginning remind the men of the simple ground rule that anything shared in the group *stays* in the group—everything's confidential. This will help the men feel safer about sharing honestly and openly in an environment of trust.

Finally, we encourage you during each meeting to allow time for prayer—conversational, short-sentence prayers expressed in honesty before God. Many men don't feel comfortable praying aloud before others, so do all you can in an understanding way to help them overcome that barrier.

What's the best way to use this workbook with my church singles group?
First, you should know that along with *Every Single Man's Battle* workbook, there is also *Every Single Woman's Battle* workbook available. This means that your single adult

ministry has all it needs to launch its members on an in-depth study of sexual purity for singles.

If your single adult ministry has gender-segregated small groups associated with it, the two workbooks are ideal curriculum for use in those small groups. In your singles group, may the men commit to the women, and the women commit to the men, to behave toward each other in all purity, as God intends.

introduction

(by Stephen Arterburn)

It is still a favorite picture of a moment I will never forget. There we were on the most beautiful beach I have ever seen, near the Great Barrier Reef of Australia. I was enjoying one of several trips I had arranged to celebrate our twentieth anniversary together, trying to mend what had been so very broken for twenty difficult years. I had thought we were making progress, and as I walked that beach with my wife, I presumed she felt as close to me as I did her. Alas, that simply was not the case. The betrayal had already occurred, and she was making plans for divorce.

It all became clear to me when we returned home. Not long after our trip to Australia, I began to suspect that something was severely wrong. Of course, something had *always* seemed wrong in our marriage—since our wedding day, we both felt we had made a big mistake.

But this time the feeling was much different. Then one day—another day frozen in my memory—a mutual friend told me of her betrayal, eventually the reason for our divorce.

I found out by cell phone as I was boarding a plane from Los Angeles to Colorado Springs, Colorado. Winging my way over the Rocky Mountains, I stared blankly out the window as my inner emotions overflowed every dike in my consciousness. Trapped on that plane, I sat strapped in with my pain, staring out the window, tears rolling down my cheeks and fear engulfing all other feelings.

I confronted her with the truth upon returning home, hoping for sorrow and a desire to work it through together, but my hopes were quickly dashed. She filed for divorce the following Monday. There would be no chance for reconciliation.

As this drama played out over the next few weeks and months, the shock was simply horrific and the pain overpowering. At first I did not want to tell anyone about anything, but the effects of my trauma quickly became obvious as I began losing weight. To those who saw me regularly, I looked thin, gaunt, and dispirited. My eyes sank deeply into dark pockets of depression, and I experienced a continual pain in the pit of my stomach as if I'd been blasted with a shotgun.

My shock and pain eventually gave way to tremendous grief. Hours were spent in tears because of the great sense of loss and betrayal I experienced. I wanted to crawl in a hole, but instead I chose to work hard at staying connected with others in spite of the grief. I protected myself with divorce-recovery meetings, Al-Anon, men's Bible studies, counseling, and a weekly meeting with a group of friends called "Couples and Steve." I connected with guys in ways I never had before. Lunches, breakfasts, and dinners were opportunities for them to help me. A true friend, Dale, was always there, encouraging me to put the shame in the past.

That choice to stay connected to others wasn't easy, as there were so many dark days. But there were peaceful days, too—days when I felt life would actually happen for me again someday. That was the hope that God was providing for me, the hope I hung on to as the pain and fear slowly subsided.

Now I'm certain the shocks didn't end at the boundaries of *my* little world. Many readers of *Every Man's Battle* will be stunned to discover that my marriage ended in 2002, and when the divorce was final in 2003, I began living the life of a single man. I had not initiated the divorce proceedings, but the single life *was* my new reality, a reality that I had to embrace and—hopefully—use to minister to others.

Fortunately for me, my board, publishers, coauthors, and friends stood with me. Many had watched for years as I tried unsuccessfully to fix my broken marriage, and they knew that my divorce was not a result of moral failure or neglect on my part. After looking diligently into the details, my board found only a tragedy—not a scandal.

I'm absolutely certain that it was not God's will that we divorce. He loves restoration, and I'm with Him on that score. But I'm just as certain that God always works everything together for good in our individual lives—and in the body of Christ—no matter how we mess up. I believe that once that door of restoration was slammed in my face, He quickly moved to Plan B to take that destruction, sin, and shame and use it for His glory.

Granted, this doesn't lessen the pain or the reality of divorce, but I still want God to use me in this. I saw a lot during my reentry into this single world, and my experiences taught me plenty about loneliness, wounds, and disconnection, and how these affect the single Christian who is committed to living a life of sexual integrity. I was also reminded once more, up close and personal, that this was no easy battle. I want to use that knowledge to help you.

It's a battle that must be engaged and won because the spiritual stakes are enormously high. I entered this new world severely wounded and vulnerable, and I wanted to be sure that I would not—in some weak moment—end up having sex with someone, which would create a new heartache and disappoint myself, God, and those who were counting on me. I was determined that I would not have sex until—if ever—I married again. I made a decision not to live a double life with a double standard. I'm hoping that you'll make the same choices.

Ever since we published *Every Man's Battle,* we've been inundated with requests for a similar resource for adult single men. No wonder. So many of America's churches are teeming with divorced singles who're clambering for answers amid the rubble of their broken hearts and shattered dreams of marriage. Senses jolted, they've joined up with their widowed and never-married brothers as single sojourners in a couple's world. They're passionately searching for answers to questions like these:

- "God couldn't possibly have meant what He said about sexual purity in the Bible, could He? Why would He create us to be sexual beings and then ask us to act asexual? It seems so unfair!"
- "I understand God's standards regarding sexual purity, but I still want some kind of sexual release. So what are my options?"
- "Does purity really make any difference in my day-to-day life? Does it really affect my intimacy with God?"
- "What do women really think of pure men? Can a romance even bloom without sex being involved?"

• "If I shut down my sexuality completely, can I be sure it'll turn on again?"

Men need the right answers if they're to move forward with God. We were created to stand in His light and to walk upright in His image as real men. We men aren't alone on this journey, of course. Our sisters are walking with us. Thankfully, our partner Shannon Ethridge, author of *Every Woman's Battle,* will help single women do that with the *Every Single Woman's Battle* workbook she's created.

What better way for everyone to get on the same page? Or, more accurately, the same *pages,* since we all need to line up and integrate our sexuality with the pages of the Bible. We need to honor women in our sexuality as Christ always did. We need to allow Christ to draw us near and heal the wounds that can trip us up in our commitment to purity. We need to arm ourselves with the attitudes of Christ toward sin:

> Therefore, since Christ suffered in his body, arm yourselves also with the same attitude, because he who has suffered in his body is done with sin. As a result, he does not live the rest of his earthly life for evil human desires, but rather for the will of God. For you have spent enough time in the past doing what the pagans choose to do—living in debauchery, *lust,* drunkenness, orgies, carousing and detestable idolatry. (1 Peter 4:1-3, emphasis added)

Are you ready to learn to walk this way as you sojourn this single pathway with your brothers and sisters in Christ?

Good. We thought so. It's time to get started!

disconnection's danger

Approaching our seaside table with a lovely new acquaintance from church, I (Steve) could hear the gentle lapping of waves on the shoreline as the magnificent amber-hued sunset arched over the Pacific Ocean. *Maybe life's not so bad after all,* I mused as we were seated and handed leather-bound menus by the maître d'.

As we perused the elegant dining choices, my date and I engaged in meaningful small talk, sharing our hopes in raising our children and our dreams of how God would use us in the future. I gazed upon the sun as it dipped toward the horizon and felt swept up in the moment. For the first time in months, the pain of my divorce seemed light-years away, and my future—whatever it would be—looked as bright as that dazzling orb descending in the western sky.

One by one the delicious courses arrived with a flourish…a crisp, deep-fried calamari as the appetizer, followed by a sumptuous spinach salad with raspberry vinaigrette dressing, and then the main course of grilled salmon topped with hollandaise sauce. *Fresh salmon heals every wound,* I chuckled to myself.

Yet just as suddenly, my bite of airy tiramisu screeched to a jarring halt halfway down the hatch as my date purred demurely, "Steve, please don't get the wrong impression of me… I'm not all God, motherhood, and apple pie, you know. I love the Bible with a deep passion, but I love the Kama Sutra with another kind of passion all my own," she said, winking coyly. "I find the positions simply fascinating, and I've thrown my whole body and soul into reading my lessons. But what I really need is to get out onto the playing field once in a while for a little practice!"

I nearly spewed my dessert coffee all over the linen-shrouded table. The only practice that was going to take place was me practicing getting out of there. First, I managed to change the subject quickly, and then, a short time later, I smiled softly and mumbled, "I really hate to run, but my food hasn't settled very well this evening. Would you mind if we called it a night?"

Perhaps you're scratching your head, wondering, *What's this Kama Sutra thing?* Well, it's all about sexual positions from an Eastern perspective, and books on the Kama Sutra have been a pretty hot topic out here on the Left Coast for quite some time. The publisher's description on Amazon.com calls it this way:

> Kama Sutra comes to us from fourth-century India. Written by a holy man, this "love scripture" has become known in the West as a "bible of sex." As such, *Kama Sutra of Sexual Positions* presents many facets of sexual embrace from many cultures where the sexual and the sacred together are the weaver of the tapestry of life.

Perhaps *now* you're gasping, *How can a Christian single be equally committed to the Kama Sutra?* I haven't the foggiest idea of how to answer that, but what I *do* know is that as I reentered the Christian single world, I was quite amazed to find two extremely common disconnections out there. My Kama Sutra story is a prime example of the first one—a disconnection from God's ways.

I've met many committed Christian singles whose faith seems to be integrated into their lives, who take a biblical approach to their work, their money, their children, whatever. But when it comes to sex, they've convinced themselves that sex is the exception to every biblical rule. They think like this:

- *God understands my sexuality—He knows my needs.*
- *Sex is just something that naturally happens between two adults who are deeply involved.*
- *I know it is wrong to have sex with a married woman, but when it comes to sex between two singles, I just don't think the Bible is so cut and dried.*
- *Anything short of sexual intercourse is okay.*
- *I know premarital sex is wrong, but so what? God will forgive me—it's under the blood!*
- *God knows that I was married. He knows I'm so used to sex that I just have to have it now.*

Such rationalizations are a deep mystery to me. After all, a *rational* mind—the mind of Christ—is normal for Christians. A rational mind keeps us safely beneath God's wings of protection and blessing. But a *rationalized* mind seems so jarring and abnormal in a Christian, and it rips a jagged breech in our sexual defense perimeters.

Look, it's time for some straight talk. As men we have an obvious vulnerability in our sexual makeup, and that's the ability of our eyes and our mind to draw vivid sexual gratification from the sensuality in the environment around us. To put it bluntly, our eyes and mind are capable of intense foreplay…we can look and lust until our engines run so far into the red zone that we may think we'd better masturbate or we'll explode. If we want to be sexually pure, we have but one choice—we either defend against such weak spots in our sexuality or we will fall to every whim of the Enemy and our flesh.

I take my defensive game seriously. Why did I change the subject so quickly from the sensuous Kama Sutra and then cut the night off early? The reason is because in that lovely, relaxed atmosphere, with the waves lapping and the stars twinkling overhead, I didn't want *my* eyes to be reminded how much *her* eyes sparkled as she spoke of her passions.

As a Christian I needed to get away—that's what real men do. I also needed to stay away. That's why I didn't go out with her again. I didn't want to tempt myself, and I didn't want thoughts of her or what the Kama Sutra might teach someone running around my mind as that second date approached.

My sexual integrity is important, and I don't apologize for it. Setting and maintaining a good defense is not dead legalism. It's wisdom. It's the mind of Christ at work. How do I know I had the mind of Christ here? Because of the truth of this Scripture:

The Word became flesh and made his dwelling among us. (John 1:14)

Jesus was the Word of God in the flesh and in fullness. Since the Bible says that we are to "flee from sexual immorality" (1 Corinthians 6:18) and since Jesus was the

Word of God in the flesh, we know exactly what He would have done in my position. Just as Jesus said in the face of one temptation, "Man does not live on bread alone" (Matthew 4:4), He would have said in the face of this temptation, "Man does not live on sex alone, but on every Word that comes from the mouth of God. So I'll flee." Jesus always obeyed Scripture, and He always had that rational mind because He was never disconnected from His Father's ways.

But unlike Jesus, men are prone to a disconnection from God's ways. We get bored with the straight life. Said another way, we quickly tire of submitting our rights to Christ. We'd rather have things our own interesting way, especially in regard to our sex lives.

The desire to control our standards and chart our own moral course can be overwhelming because our sexuality is so tightly tied to our male ego. We give God a say on a few things while retaining our veto power in case the road gets too narrow. No wonder I get e-mails like this so often:

> I now see all the reasons why my attempts for "sexual sobriety" have failed. I had said to myself many times, *I'll give up pornography, but not masturbation* or *I'll give up everything but checking out women.*

Note his exercise of the line-item veto, a veto that allows his sexual defenses to be compromised through a breech that remains in his eyes and mind. It is always the line-item veto that spawns rationalization's drift from God's *ways,* and over the long haul, our compromised defenses spawn a distance from God *Himself.*

In *Every Man's Battle* I (Fred) described this veil of distance and how it choked my ability to pray and to freely worship God. Steve and I then spent most of the book defining practical defense strategies to create protection against that vulnerability of our eyes and mind in our sexual makeup.

If you are to remain sexually pure as a single man, you must shore up this weakness with everything you've got, and you must also avoid any disconnection from God's ways that opens a breech into your heart. But we have a second huge vulnerability in our sexual makeup that we didn't cover in *Every Man's Battle,* and it's this: the Enemy uses a second form of disconnection—a disconnection from people—to open another broad breech in our sexual defenses.

It's quite obvious why Satan wants you to get disconnected from God's ways: once you're off the reservation, he knows that your very own eyes and mind will work against you in this fight for purity.

But why would he want you disconnected from people? He knows this second vulnerability works the same way—if he can keep you disconnected from others, your own sexual makeup plays right into his hands. It's no exaggeration to say that for single men this second form of disconnection is practically as dangerous to your sexual purity as a disconnection from God's ways.

What does this vulnerability look like? By nature, we men get our physical intimacy tanks filled most satisfactorily from what we do just prior to and during intercourse. Essentially, it is our native language of intimacy, the way we naturally long to share it. (Women, on the other hand, share their intimacy in talking, sharing, hugging, and touching. Her sexual triggers, by nature, are more relational.)

If you've ever wondered why we tend to push so hard against the sexual boundaries of our girlfriends when we're dating, it's not because we're godless pigs—it's because we're longing to express our hearts in our own innate language of love.

But that presents a couple of problems. First, we aren't supposed to use this native language anywhere else but within our marital relationship. Even more troubling is that nearly all of the body's most powerful chemicals are involved in that wash of pleasure chemicals that flood the brain's limbic centers during an orgasm. This means that it's pretty easy for men to confuse the passage of true intimacy with the feelings they experience during premarital sex and even those associated with porn and masturbation. The following e-mail from a reader states this point well:

> What do I get with porn? I like how naked women look in the pictures. They look so seductive, so sexy, and they are willing to show you all they've got. They are there to please me, and I don't have to give anything in

return. I can take whatever I want, when I want, and how I want through masturbation.

The bottom line is this: the pleasure chemicals involved in porn and masturbation are a seductively powerful substitute for reality. First of all, an orgasm produces a strong sense of manhood in a guy. He feels dominant and strong at the moment of release, even though the sensation is fleeting. Second, he also feels a strong sense of intimate connection with another human being at that moment, even though the experience is over in a flash.

For a lonely and disconnected man, that sense of manhood and intimate connection is an extremely potent draw, which explains why porn and masturbation shine like a pan of fool's gold to his eyes. What a guy can't get through a real sexual encounter, he believes he can get through looking at porn and ejaculating, because it feels good and provides many of the same feelings as the real thing.

It isn't long before self-stimulation becomes the medicating drug of choice for our pain, and masturbation is far easier to choose over drugs and alcohol because it doesn't just get us high. A real-time orgasm feels like real intimacy, if only for a moment.

Now how does all this play into Satan's hands? Wounds and isolation have always been the open door to this trap, and you surely don't have to be divorced to know what we're talking about. Wounds that form a hole in our heart can launch us toward sexual sin, and our sexual makeup sets us up to fall. My dad wounded me deeply, especially when I was playing quarterback on my high-school football team. On the mornings after our Friday-night games, Dad delivered horrible verbal blitzes about every mistake I had made. After one tirade, I got so nauseous that I took off my cap and vomited into it. This wounded me deeply and left me lonely and aching.

Do you remember the primary way guys give and receive intimacy? That's right, through the acts just prior to and during intercourse. What can give guys that feeling of intimacy, that feeling of love and acceptance? Right again—the always smiling, always available, and always unclothed girls of cyberspace. They never reject you, and they always offer you everything they've got while asking nothing in return.

Without that connection with our fathers and that acceptance as men, we are very vulnerable to sexual sin during our teen years and beyond. Orgasmic relief is the medication of our pain. And once this becomes our crutch in our crippled interpersonal life, we'll drag that crutch right into our adult years. It happens to many of us simply because of our sexual makeup.

The deepest wound my dad ever inflicted on me was his divorce. As I've said, masturbation is a way young men can salve deep insecurity or psychological pain, and nothing delivers a load of pain quite like divorce.

Sexual sin flourishes in the wake of bad or broken family relationships. The splintering effects of divorce (or parental death) shatter our worlds. Teens, rather than feeling accepted and cherished by their parents, feel as though they've been cast aside. They spend their lives searching for love and meaning, when it should have been provided in the home by a loving mother and a loving father.

Patrick Middleton, a good friend and a gifted addictions counselor, recently told me, "I deal with a lot of adult men, and it never fails that the men with the deeper sexual issues also have uninvolved or missing fathers. Their sexual issues are directly and severely impacted by their dad's failures as a father."

Perhaps you've felt the pain in your past family relationships, or perhaps your pain stems from a more recent family disruption through your own divorce, like mine (Steve). The desire to become close to *somebody* can also drive you quickly into the arms of cyberspace or short-term sexual relationships with women. Rather than turn to God, you truly can begin looking for love in all the wrong places, hoping for something, anything, to take the place of that loss.

Obviously this is where our maleness works against us. Just think about my (Steve's) story for a minute. I didn't want a divorce, but when it happened, my soul was flooded by shame and alienation. Since it seemed to me that my life was basically over, I wanted to crawl into a hole. I was certain I would never get to write books again and that Christians everywhere would reject me. Hurt and wounded, it was tempting to latch on to the first life preserver that floated by, and the false intimacy of porn and masturbation was only a mouse-click away. For any of us, an orgasmic surge of power and virility can seem to be just what the doctor might order for wounds like ours. I determined with God's help that porn and masturbation would not be part of my single life. I know they don't have to be part of yours or any single man's life.

An Inner Focus—and More Isolation

By now you should understand that masturbation is an implosion of sexual pleasure that focuses a guy further and further into himself. But the genuine need for interpersonal intimacy simply cannot be met by self-seeking sexual activity. It's like slaking your parched thirst with salt water. A sip can satisfy for a moment, but the eventual results are disastrous. If you masturbate to "fix" your feelings of insecurity and isolation, then masturbation just adds to your loneliness, because you're not receiving true intimacy when you do the act.

If you asked a woman to explain porn's potent draw to us, she'd cite the sex appeal of limitless free and frisky women to the male eyes and mind. But we know there are more complex factors at work here. Porn provides an instant soothing to emotional stress, and easy access to Internet porn makes it difficult to wean men away from their emotional dependence on it.

Remember, your sexuality is a primary communication line for transmitting and receiving intimacy. When that line goes down, your emotional life shrivels, and the effects upon marriage are disastrous.

Tragically, porn's first major blow does exactly this—decoupling sex entirely from the communication of intimacy. Over time, sexual *intensity* will replace *intimacy* as your primary focus of sex. This is where significant damage to our sexuality begins.

How in the world does this happen? Like a germ using a cell's own DNA to reproduce, porn and masturbation use a man's own hardwiring to destroy itself. It all starts innocently enough, with the eyes feasting naturally on the sexual images, just as they were created to do. The orgasmic chemical responses hit the pleasure centers like a dream—again, just as they were created to do. Then the addictive component develops, which will keep someone coming back for more porn and masturbation. Once that happens, he's hooked, and looking at porn becomes part of his life.

It is here where porn initiates a cataclysmic feedback loop in our hardwiring. Pornography's affect on the brain is Pavlovian, and each orgasm is a huge reenforcer.

Now if your hardwiring is normal, as God created it, at the right time your focus will not be on yourself but on your future wife and her pleasure. Your orgasms will happen with her, and because of that, you will associate your orgasms with your wife: her kiss, her scent, her body. Because of that reinforcement, that is what will turn you on over time and will keep you fascinated with the wife of your youth.

If you open your boundaries to endless transgressions by the harems of cyber-space, however, your sexual proclivities and tastes will go in other directions. That won't be good for you…or your future wife.

Worse, your hardwiring will morph and bring in an unnatural obsession with looking at women rather than interacting with them. It will bring an attitude that objectifies women and rates them by size, shape, and harmony of body parts. And the morphing? The visual side of your sexual hardwiring gets supersized, creating an obsession with visual stimulation (for instance, the bigger the breasts the better) while the transmission-of-intimacy side ("I so love your soul, honey") shrivels away.

Once intensity takes the place of intimacy, and intimacy is then decoupled from sex, the sexual high is the end in itself. As we said, the transmitters get fried, which means the future marriage bed is cooked before you get started. Your souls and spirits won't be meeting in bed…only the bodies will be connecting. And more often than not, the gentle affection and climactic touch that your wife needs will no longer hold any interest for you. Your attitude will go something like this: *All aboard my one-way express to Sex City! Grab what you can, honey, but I'm the one who counts! Pour the fuel into my engines, and don't you dare tap on the brakes.*

Where your natural hardware would have prompted you to initiate normal inti-mate connections with your wife, now it will just prod you for another intense orgas-mic hit, sometimes with your wife, sometimes with the computer. The computer sex may be intense, but it's always soulless and cold, just like sex might be with your wife. As you both drift to sleep afterward, she's still lonely, and you've gotten nothing but high. *What's intimacy got to do with it?*

Since I (Steve) have reentered the single world, I've met many, many men with almost an aversion to getting involved with women. These guys have essentially received their sex education on the Internet and find no reason—or deeply desired need—to pursue an actual woman. They prefer to stay in their apartments and have sex with themselves within the harems of cyberspace. These guys have been so brainwashed by Internet porn that they're unwilling to go through the struggle, pain, and effort to develop a relationship with a real live woman.

In many ways a kind of porn creep takes over. Jacob, a Christian twentysomething, told us that after watching porn videos for a couple of years, he met a beautiful woman at work. She was sexually loose and agreed to join him for a weekend of sex at a resort. They acted out what both had viewed in pornography. When it was over, Jacob said, "I felt nothing."

Jacob sought to find the same intensity he'd felt watching the videos, but he didn't find it with a real woman, even in a glorious resort hotel room, because she couldn't take him where his own hands and fantasies could. Porn and masturbation will creep in and take over your sexual makeup, eventually frying everything to a crisp.

Guys depending upon porn, masturbation, and premarital sex *will* have trouble forming healthy relationships with women and with their future wives and, perhaps surprisingly, *will* even have trouble forming a few healthy relationships with guys, because of the deep pools of guilt and shame they're drowning in.

If you're feeling lonely and disconnected, that is a red flag to get up and get moving toward others *today* in order to close that breech in your defenses.

getting connected
without hooking up

"Single men should not live alone," said Mason, a thirtysomething single pastor who has never married—and still lives alone. "I guess I shouldn't be dogmatic about it because I've been living by myself for a number of years, but I'm starting to wonder if single guys should really live all by themselves. After all, the apostle Paul was single and strong as anyone spiritually, yet he always traveled with other men. Living with guys provides a natural accountability, a natural hook to reality that could stop a guy's mind from running away with itself sexually. Having roommates would also remind guys like me that we're part of something bigger in life, and that our decisions really do affect the people around us."

It was apparent that Mason had given a lot of thought to life as a single. Since he hadn't married in his twenties, did he expect to remain single a long time? "Probably, for a couple of reasons," he replied. "Look, I love my freedom to serve the Lord. If an inner-city student calls me at three in the morning and says he's in trouble, I jump in the car and go. But if I were married, I would be leaving my wife in the middle of the night, so there would be ramifications for both of us in leaving her. Because of that, I'd prefer to stay single for now from a ministry standpoint. There's another reason, and it's because I personally don't believe that marriage makes the battle for sexual purity much easier."

Marriage doesn't make the battle for sexual purity easier? What did he mean by that?

The young pastor explained that as a pastor he does a lot of marital counseling, and after years of wrestling with couples and their issues, he honestly believes that being single is far easier than being married. For instance, after all the times he's heard husbands tell him how their wives make themselves sexually unavailable, he thinks it's easier for a single man to stay sexually pure than a married one. "After all," he reasons,

"I don't have a nude lady walking in and out of the shower at my place, or one who prances around in lingerie at bedtime with every intention of shutting me off because she's thinking, *Why should I have sex with him? I just don't feel like it these days.*"

But Mason remains conflicted. "While there's no question in my mind that it's good for a man to be single, just as Paul said, it's not good for that man to be alone, and there lies the conundrum."

As Mason shared his thoughts, I (Fred) mused on the ministry of the apostle Paul, who preferred being single for some of the same reasons Mason mentioned (see 1 Corinthians 7:32-35). Yet as a diligent student of the Scriptures, Paul could never forget that God declared that it is not good for man to be alone (see Genesis 2:18). Perhaps that is one reason Paul chose to travel with a group of guys throughout his ministry.

My mind ran further along these lines when Mason uttered the phrase, "Living with guys provides a natural accountability," which triggered a memory of a story we shared in *Every Man's Battle:*

> Sid races home by 4 p.m. every summer day. That's when his neighbor
> Angela sunbathes right outside his window. "At four o'clock, she lies out
> in a bikini, and she doesn't know I can see her. I can gaze to my heart's
> content. She's so sexy I can hardly stand it, and I masturbate every day
> I see her."

As we build more connection into our lives, we are building protective defenses in our battle for purity. Obviously Sid couldn't play this dark afternoon game if there was a possibility that one of his roommates could walk in on him at any time.

This was hitting closer to home now. I (Fred) thought back to the torturous nights I spent in hotels across Iowa and South Dakota when I was traveling in sales. I *dreaded* these hotels, just as Wally, another businessman and frequent traveler, told us. "I always eat a long, leisurely supper," he said, "stalling before returning to my room because I know what's coming. Before too long I have the TV remote in my hand. I tell myself it'll only be for a minute, but I know I'm lying. I know what I really want. I'm hoping to catch a little sex scene or two as I search the channels. I tell myself that I'll only watch for a while, or that I'll stop before I get carried away. But then my motor gets going and I lust for more, sometimes even turning to the hotel's 'adult channel.'

"The RPMs get going so high I have to do something, or it feels like my engine will blow. So I masturbate. On a few occasions I fought it, but if I did that, later on, when I turned the lights out, my mind was flooded with lustful thoughts and desires. That's when I would stare wide-eyed at the ceiling, seeing nothing but literally feeling the bombardment, the throbbing desire. There was no way I could fall sleep; that's how much it was killing me. I would say to myself, 'Okay, if I masturbate, I'll have some peace, and I can finally get to sleep.' So I did what came naturally, and you know what? The guilt was so strong I *still* couldn't get to sleep anyway. I would wake up totally exhausted in the morning."

Single men can face these temptations *every* night if they don't have roommates to help fill the time, and the natural accountability that comes with a shared apartment can be a huge ally in the fight, which is one good reason for getting and staying connected with one or more single guy, housemates.

STRATEGIES TO CONSIDER

But the value of connection stretches well beyond the basics of natural accountability. When Steve shared his story about his date with the comely Kama Sutra disciple, I (Fred) remembered my earlier days of premarital sexual activity. "Steve," I blurted, "when I was younger, if a woman had talked about wanting to try out some sexual positions with me, those mental images would have been frozen in my mind. I would have lustfully returned to them countless times over the new few days and surely would have wanted to personally try those new positions with her—or slipped into masturbation over it all."

When my writing partner agreed with me, I posed this question. "Steve, you're single now. How have you managed to keep from thinking about what she said? Are you simply taking the thoughts captive and dumping them?" We both knew that the idea of taking thoughts captive and getting rid of them through the Holy Spirit was something we wrote about in *Every Man's Battle*.

"Well, that did play a role," Steve conceded. "But the big thing is that I had people to talk to. Right away I told my friends John and Henry about that conversation with her—what happened, what I felt inside sexually when she said it, and what I did to flee the situation. As a single guy I find that having somebody to talk to about things like that prevents the secret, lustful thoughts from building up inside. You laugh about it, talk about it, pray about it together—anyway, the whole thing kind of diffuses in the process. Those thoughts did not come to mind very often at all, but when they did, I would bounce my mind the way we bounce our eyes. I would simply focus on something else. Sometimes I would start singing the first line of a song, and by the time I was at the end of that line the thought was gone. Eventually those thoughts stopped coming as soon as I talked to someone about it."

I whistled in admiration, but then Steve had a question for me.

"Fred, I'll bet that when you were younger and dealing with those same kinds of thoughts, you didn't have Christian men in your life to share these things with. If you had, maybe some of those things you went through wouldn't have happened."

"You're probably right," I responded wistfully. "So you're saying that talking with John and Henry helps keep you on the straight and narrow?"

"So far, so good," he replied. "They're also going to ask if I have called her back and asked her out again in some weak moment, just to keep me honest. They've both said that they would jump all over me if I did that."

Steve's on the right track. The connection of friendship provides another form of natural accountability, a hedge against hypocrisy in our actions. Like Steve, Danny consciously builds this accountability into his life because he cares about his purity:

> Because I'm single, I tell every guy that I know about my standards for
> dating women. The way I see things, my standards are easier to keep if the
> guys know what they are. That way, if I mess up, I figure that every guy in

town would hear about it sooner or later and let me know about it. I have made conscious choices like this to set me apart from "average" Christian guys who never quite stay pure. I really want to do God's perfect will, and I've come to believe that you have to love God's ways enough to sacrifice for them.

If you're thinking, *Look, I can do this on my own!* I sure understand the sentiment. I (Fred) grew up loving action heroes like Clint Eastwood, Sylvester Stallone, and Arnold Schwarzenegger, and as a guy, I'm sure you'd love to be able to grab this thing by the throat and smash it on your own. Besides, there is no doubt that ultimately it's crucial to form your own strong internal defenses that require no one else's presence, especially since our culture is so sexually wild and sick.

It's like in the *Star Trek* series, where a Class-M planet is one whose environment is like earth's. A Class-M planet isn't hostile to human life, and men can move about such planets without spacesuits. Here on earth, parents often spend all their time creating Class-M environments in their homes…employing filters and defenses and bubbles to create a nonhostile environment for their kids. But what happens when those young graduates leave these friendly confines? When my son Jasen was launched, he splashed down at Iowa State University, and we knew this going in: ISU was no Class-M planet! Some have questioned our wisdom in not sending our son to a Class-M Christian college, but Jasen knew that he had what he needed to survive in such a hostile environment.

That's good because let's face it: at some point, nearly all men will explore a hostile planet or two as they travel through their college and career galaxies. That's why they need spacesuits and *internal* filters to protect them from these hostile environments and why each of us must be man enough to step up and build these internal defenses into our lives.

But even if you have these filters firmly in place, like Jasen does, it would be foolish to dismiss your other defenses—defenses like having a layering of male friends surrounding you and who have connected with you so that you can fight shoulder to shoulder. I can assure you that while Jasen is very pure and strong in his internal convictions, he knows that he should still surround himself with three Christian roommates as well.

Maybe you've overlooked the importance of surrounding yourself with godly men. Maybe you think you have everything under control. If so, let me remind you that you have a weak spot in your sexuality that will always be open to attack by disconnection, no matter how strong your internal defenses feel today.

You see, it's not just the natural accountability in these relationships that gives connection its power. It's the intimacy itself. You may not think you need the accountability in order to stand, but I can assure you, you do need the intimacy. It's because intimacy itself has a power to free you.

That's why connection is not so much about accountability as it's about a genuine intimacy. Most men fall because they have little true intimacy and connection in their lives, and they seek the false intimacy of porn and masturbation to make up for it. When they want out later on, it's not only hard to kick the chemical highs physically, it's also hard to kick the emotional dependency they have upon the false feelings of intimacy that come with it all. Granted, those feelings are always false and fleeting, but if that's all they've had because of the disconnection in their lives, they'll miss it a lot when it goes.

While genuine intimacy is able to protect you from falling into sexual sin in the first place, the power of interpersonal relationships is also so potent that it can sometimes break the power of an existing masturbation cycle practically on its own, turning things around and bringing an early, unexpected end to the battle. Rich found this to be true in his life:

> I felt very insecure as a child. Dad wasn't a cold person, but he was distant because he worked a lot, so I bonded closely with a domineering, legalistic mother. Consequently, I never really felt like one of the guys. At school, I wasn't much of an athlete, so I played in the band. On top off that, my classmates tormented me, so I turned to masturbation to cope.

My porn and masturbation habits were never really about sex. They were about medicating pain and seeking *emotional intimacy....* Masturbation was just my medication of choice.... But you know what eventually seemed to help the most in breaking this cycle of porn? It turned out to be my best friend, Eric, who really turned the tide for me. He was the first guy who truly accepted me as a man and as a friend. He affirmed my masculinity through our hiking adventures and our talks. Sometimes I think that a strong, masculine friend was all I needed.

Men need to be accepted as men, and this man found freedom through the heart of a friend. This is the very reason accountability groups can be so vital in this battle. It's not just that you have friends looking over your shoulder, it's that the true intimacy of friendship and acceptance actually heals the underlying wounds so that the false intimacy of masturbation and porn is no longer needed as a pain-killing medication.

POWER OF ACCOUNTABILITY

Christian men are teaming up as bands of brothers in this fight. Sure, they've had to humble themselves by opening up to each other, but there has never been a time that has been easier to do that than today. Men all around the country are talking about the most embarrassing things—including masturbation—and finding victory as they connect with others on these deeper issues.

If we are vulnerable and open to taking a risk with our brothers, we are never doomed to fail or to live a life of loneliness and isolation. Jesus wants us to take His weapons and fight shoulder to shoulder with our brothers:

Be prepared. You're up against far more than you can handle on your own. Take all the help you can get, every weapon God has issued, so that when it's all over but the shouting you'll still be on your feet. Truth, righteousness, peace, faith, and salvation are more than words. Learn how to apply them. You'll need them throughout your life. God's Word is an *indispensable* weapon. In the same way, prayer is essential in this ongoing warfare. Pray hard and long. Pray for your brothers and sisters. Keep your eyes open. Keep each other's spirits up so that no one falls behind or drops out. (Ephesians 6:13-18, MSG)

We aren't called to hide our lust from our brothers or to manage our lust on our own. We're called to march out resolutely and to kill our lust—together. Choose up teams and choose your weapons well. Then go out and win.

OUR CONNECTION WITH WOMEN

Perhaps you're wondering, *I understand that I need to get connected with guys now, but does that mean I can't connect with women, too?* That's a great question, and of course you should connect with women. But you need to be wise.

For the first six months after my marriage ended, I (Steve) chose not to even talk to those of the opposite sex—in a fun, guy-enjoying-girl kind of way—and that turned out to be a good decision. I would tell anyone who's divorced that you absolutely must wait a certain amount of time after the marriage has ended before you jump feet first into the singles world of dating. You need to wait before you get involved with someone else, even though you may *feel* otherwise. Don't trust your feelings…trust what others tell you or what you may already know yourself—that you first need to take the time to grow and connect with people of the same sex.

As I said earlier, when I was divorced I wanted to crawl in a hole, and if you're in my situation, you'll be hurting severely. If you get involved in dating too quickly, you'll tend to latch on to the first person who comes along. They don't call it "on the rebound" for nothing.

I understand that perhaps it was never your intent to reenter the single world. I know how that feels. Perhaps for the last five years you had no more than a roommate relationship with your wife—lots of clashes and little sex or intimacy. Now that the divorce decree is final, you want to move on with your life and find a woman sooner rather than later. If that's the way you're thinking, I urge you to back off a bit.

No matter how you rationalize it, you are reentering the single world patched up and using crutches, so you need to get your heart settled before dating again. And even when you do begin dating, you need to do it differently that you ever did before. You need to seek friendship first and leave romantic connections out of the loop for some time.

My friends John and Henry—actually, they're my radio partners John Townsend and Henry Cloud on the New Life Live! program—have been keeping me company in my foxhole. Doing the radio program with them has given me the opportunity to speak with them during the breaks about my new life as a single man. I've asked for their advice, and they've provided me with guidelines on how to make healthy decisions. One of the things they suggested was to make one very important promise to them: before I settled on one person to enter into a significant relationship with someday, I had to get to know and even date a good number of different people first.

You may be scratching your head and wondering how this advice squares with that given in books like *I Kissed Dating Goodbye* in which Joshua Harris taught against serial dating—a series of relationships where both parties give away serious portions of their hearts before the breakup.

That's not at all what John and Henry had in mind when they offered that advice. All three of us agree that practice relationships are a recipe for pain and disaster. That's why they proposed that I go out on some one-night, friend-type dates just for the sake of hanging out with another human being and enjoying her as a person. *Then* I could get more serious.

That would give the pain a chance to subside and get me on an even keel so that I needn't approach any date with an air of desperation. The last thing they wanted was for me to attach myself too tightly to someone prematurely.

John and Henry also recommended that I double date for a vast majority of those early dates. That would give me some solid protection while I learned to connect with women again.

Of course, there is some danger in this approach, because you can find yourself sitting across the table from a woman basically offering herself for an evening of sexual fun (like my Kama Sutra gal). But I was able to take that situation and learn from it—like ask for the check and get out of there! The rest of the time my dates have been positive experiences, and we really connected as people.

In fact, I think John and Henry are on to something (Henry's even written a book on the topic, *How to Get a Date Worth Keeping*). I'm finding that being a single man in this day and age can be a lot of fun. There are far more ways to meet people than ever before, whether it's through a Christian dating service or through singles groups at church. And as opposed to my earlier days in high school and college, this time around, I have dates for the right reasons.

a sexual sabbatical

In this chapter I (Fred) want to speak candidly to men who have had sexual experience inside or outside of marriage. If you are not sexually experienced, this interval will be *helpful,* so I want you to read carefully. However, my primary focus here is on the man who may think he *deserves* sex.

Too many singles believe that once the sexual genie has been let out of the bottle in marriage, it's ridiculous to try to put it back in. *God couldn't possibly have meant what He said about sexual purity in the Bible,* they reason. *He understands my needs, and even if He doesn't, He'll forgive me! Besides, I'm used to having sex, so how can He expect to shut off that spigot? I want it.*

If some—or all—of those thoughts have crossed your mind, then you'll do well to note how Christ spoke against the early church at Ephesus:

> Yet I hold this against you: You have forsaken your first love. Remember
> the height from which you have fallen! Repent and do the things you did
> at first. If you do not repent, I will come to you and remove your lampstand
> from its place. But you have this in your favor: You hate the practices of the
> Nicolaitans, which I also hate. (Revelation 2:4-6)

The Nicolaitans believed their spiritual liberty gave them leeway to practice sexual immorality, and Jesus praised Ephesus for hating that. What about you? Do you hate the practices of the Nicolaitans? If you've already justified in your mind that it's fine to get your next date into bed, Christ has a hard warning for you: *You've fallen even further than the Ephesians! You have not only forsaken your first love, but you also love the things I hate.*

God despises the very sexual practices that you love. He was against the Nicolaitans, and if you persist in having premarital sex, then He'll be against you as well.

You know, the Nicolaitans probably believed that they were good, solid Christians too. But the apostle John told such men that if anyone loves the world—the cravings of sinful man, the lust of his eyes—the love of the Father is not in him (see 1 John 2:15).

So what does it mean when you firmly assert, *I'm used to having sex and I'm going to have it?* Either you aren't saved or you're incredibly deceived. The apostle Paul warned you to watch for such great deception in yourself:

> No immoral, impure or greedy person—such a man is an idolater—has any inheritance in the kingdom of Christ and of God. Let no one deceive you with empty words, for because of such things God's wrath comes on those who are disobedient. Therefore do not be partners with them. (Ephesians 5:5-7)

Did you notice that he called you an idolater? In Romans 16:10, Paul called his friend Apelles "tested and approved in Christ." Are you tested and approved in Christ, or have you been deceived with empty words?

It's an incredibly important question, considering that our hearts are deceitful (see Jeremiah 17:9) and easily fooled. Jesus told us ahead of time that there would be many who think they are Christians when they are actually not (see Matthew 7:21-23). He also told us that He would allow false believers to grow up and live among those that are truly His until the final day (see Matthew 13:24-30).

The deceptive spirit of the Nicolaitans is still around these days, though it's now practicing under a new name—the postmodern philosophies that claim nobody has a monopoly on the truth. While few professing Christians openly reject absolute truth, many happily mix Christ's grace into this no-one-has-a-monopoly philosophy to stir up a certifiably and despicably Nicolaitan brew, easily recognized in statements like:

- "I'm doing it all—the sex, the masturbation—in my own home, and it isn't affecting others."

- "What I'm doing certainly isn't hurting my relationship with God, because He loves me no matter what."

Sound familiar? Look, there's no such thing as doing something alone in your own home. He is always there with you, and so it always affects at least the Lord. While His *love* for you will never be affected, your actions will affect your *intimacy* with Him. You'll feel further away, and your oneness with Him will fade. The scary thing is that if you've passed out spiritually from swilling this Nicolaitan brew, you might not even *notice* that there's a gulf between you and the Lord. If this is the case in your life, the apostle Paul is shaking you:

> Wake up from your slumber.... Let us put aside the deeds of darkness and put on the armor of light. Let us behave decently...not in sexual immorality.... Rather, clothe yourselves with the Lord Jesus Christ, and do not think about how to gratify the desires of the sinful nature. (Romans 13:11-14)

When Paul exhorts you to clothe yourself with the Lord Jesus Christ, he's asking you to display outwardly what has already taken place inwardly—if it has—by practicing all the virtues associated with Christ.

Now don't get me wrong. I (Fred) am not talking so much about your *success* in the battle for purity as I am about your *heart*. God is no grouch. In fact, I've never joined up with a kinder friend in any sport or battle, and without a doubt, the one thing that impressed me most during my own battle for purity was His heart.

He was so quick to encourage me to get back up again that it was almost as if He didn't care that I'd stumbled. As long as I hadn't quit fighting His fight, even though the tide of battle ebbed and flowed, He was with me from start to finish. He was my daddy, and He believed in me because I was His son. He knew the power I had inside of me to win—He Himself had placed it there the evening I was saved. He knew what I'd grow up to be if I'd just turn toward His ways and turn away from my flesh.

None of this is about your perfection or my perfection but rather accepting *His* perfection as your only call, your only aim. And it's about your precious love for Him:

> The person who knows my commandments and keeps them, that's who
> loves me. And the person who loves me will be loved by my Father, and I
> will love him and make myself plain to him. (John 14:21, MSG)

Our call to purity has always been about relationship. That's why He made us, and that's why He sent His Son, that we might walk with Him in the garden once again in the cool of the day, shoulder to shoulder, heart to heart. He aches for our love and our oneness with Him.

But the man with the haughty sexual spirit has placed his sexual pleasure on the throne of his heart. These sex-sated guys are described in the Bible like this: "With eyes full of adultery, they never stop sinning; they seduce the unstable" (2 Peter 2:14), and guys on the make "worm their way into homes and gain control over weak-willed women, who are loaded down with sins and are swayed by all kinds of evil desires, always learning but never able to acknowledge the truth" (2 Timothy 3:6-7).

This could be you. Are you always learning about Christ but never able to acknowledge His truth as the center of your sexual life? Are you a man after God's own heart, or a man after satisfying your own sexual urges? Choose your destiny:

> Now fear the LORD and serve him with all faithfulness. Throw away the
> gods your forefathers worshiped…and serve the LORD. (Joshua 24:14)

I (Fred) made that choice. My forefathers—my father and both grandfathers—wormed their way into many homes and beds, and all three loved porn throughout their lives, whether they were married or single. I once joined them in worshiping these gods, but not anymore. I've thrown them away.

What will *you* do? As you're deciding, consider my paraphrase of Joshua 24:15: "If serving the Lord sexually seems undesirable to you, then choose for yourselves this day whom you *will* serve, whether the gods of your forefathers, or the sensual gods of the Americans, in whose land you are living. But as for me and my body, we will serve the Lord."

A COVENANT WITH THE EYES

I (Steve) am with Fred. I wanted to save sex for remarriage because it was the right thing to do and because sexual integrity can keep the intimate connection with God open and allow it to grow deeper.

In *Every Man's Battle,* Fred said that when he made a covenant—like Job did—not to look lustfully with his eyes, he felt a new light and lightness in his soul. When Fred's sexual sin—which had brought a darkness so deep and smothering—vanished, the difference was so real he could practically touch it. Fred felt loved and approved by God.

Garrett's story paints a similar picture:

> I could barely believe what happened after I starting guarding my eyes! I'd been in ministerial studies for a year and a half already, so you have to know that I was reading my Bible plenty. I was praying a lot too.
>
> But when I started bouncing my eyes, and the lust rolled away, it was as if the Bible opened up like a blue sky before me after a really dark night. Bouncing my eyes really helped me read and understand my Bible better.
>
> And I've noticed an interesting thing: when I read my Bible less and don't stay close to the Word, it's harder to bounce my eyes. They really go hand in hand, and one can't be done very well without the other.
>
> As for my prayer times—my oh my. I used to get lustful thoughts popping up all the time during prayer. But now that my eyes are protected, it doesn't happen, so prayer has become so much deeper and uninterrupted. Worshiping God is better as well. Now I feel free to express my heart to God. Before, I didn't have the freedom to express my love to God, probably because I was too involved in impure thoughts and stuff.

That deeper connection with God is the end game regarding sexual purity for all of us, and this truth has been especially meaningful to me when my painful divorce tumbled me into survival mode. Those days brought to mind that age-old mantra of the lost hiker or the marooned sea captain: survival is the first order of business. Like the lost and marooned, when our relationships are broken, our first instinct is the same—to grab at anything with survival promise. But in our case that first instinct would be wrong, because for the wounded Christian single, survival—which could mean looking for a date or another porn site—is *not* our first order of business. Revival is.

In fact, spiritual revival is the first order of business for *all* singles, whether you're wounded or not. Our single years are not only a time to connect with other people, but it can be a time to connect deeply with God like none other, because, like Paul said, "An unmarried man is concerned about the Lord's affairs—how he can please the Lord. But a married man is concerned about the affairs of this world—how he can please his wife—and his interests are divided.… I am saying this for your own good, not to restrict you, but that you may live in a right way in *undivided devotion* to the Lord" (1 Corinthians 7:32-35, emphasis added).

Our *sexual* revival must also be our first order of business during our single years, as there is no better time to maintain or reboot our sexual hard drive to God's original specs. In *Every Man's Battle,* I (Fred) told of a song popular during my senior year of college in which the singer mourned about trying to remember how it used to feel when a kiss was something special. The lyrics from the song resonated with me because, at that point in my life, a kiss meant nothing. Kissing was a joyless prerequisite on the path to intercourse.

My heavy use of porn and women had decoupled sex entirely from the communication of intimacy, just as we said earlier. During that time sexual *intensity* had replaced *intimacy* as my primary focus of sex. Something was deeply wrong, but I ignored any second thoughts about using women for my sexual pleasure, whether in porn or in person. Like so many of us, I had gotten to the point where *looking* at women was more important than *interacting* with them, objectifying them and rating them by size, shape, and harmony of body parts. My sexual hard drive was damaged.

This same damage explains why it's been so novel for me (Steve) to hang out with or date a number of women simply for the fun of human connection without the sexual undertones of desire. That's not the way I looked at women back when I was in college. My mind-set was the opposite of God's specific direction:

> Treat…older women as mothers, and younger women as sisters, with
> absolute purity. (1 Timothy 5:1-2)

I looked at this verse with a fresh set of eyes ever since my divorce. For me to treat women "with absolute purity," I needed a sexual revival of sorts—a new way of thinking this time around the single track. Since I could not have sexual revival if I'm out looking for sex all the time, I made a decision: I went on a sexual sabbatical.

In the workplace sabbaticals are a time of refreshment, a time to lay aside the busyness and get away from the ringing telephones to pursue something deeper in our hearts or the world around us. Sabbaticals are a time to refresh and renew while seeking richer purposes. We don't quit our careers…we simply stop out for a while.

A sexual sabbatical can be similar. We view this type of sabbatical as a time to downplay our natural sexual drives and passions while we pursue a deeper connection with God. Sure, the sexual side is still there. We've simply determined to direct our attention and energy to God. We use this period of sexual inactivity to cut away every hint of immorality and all of porn's medications to focus upon actual healing and depth in God.

A sexual revival can be a springboard to full spiritual revival. No matter how close you are to God, the question is clear: How much closer do you want to be? Would it be this close?

> Love the Lord your God with all your heart and with all your soul and with
> all your mind and with all your strength. (Mark 12:30)

Be honest with yourself: have you ever really loved God with all your heart? We're not talking about walking around with a Bible in your hand or playing in the worship band or going on a missions trip every summer. What we're asking is this:

- Have you ever really been madly, passionately in love with Jesus?
- When was the last time you felt so close to the Lord that you could almost feel His passion for the lost?
- Have you ever sobbed in prayer for the lost? your church? your pastor?

I (Fred) once heard evangelist Michael Brown say, "I once saw my single years as a kind of lonely exile, and so I was especially focused on having something to do with my friends on Friday and Saturday nights. But sometimes I'd call them and learn, one by one, that they had other plans. My stomach churned with each successive phone call as it became clear that I'd have nothing to do and no place to go.

"One night I heard God whisper, *Why not spend the evening with Me? I've got nothing going tonight.* It had never occurred to me that perhaps God had arranged for my friends to be busy so that I could spend some time with Him. That's exactly what I did, and I got my Bible and worship tapes out and experienced some of the most intimate, precious times I've ever known. From that time forward I never panicked when my friends were busy on the weekends. I'd just climb up into His arms and spend the evening with Him."

Intimate passion for Jesus comes from spending deep time alone with Him. This kind of passion may sound foreign to you, and many Christians never take the time to find it. But how about starting with an hour of prayer and worship, just you and Jesus?

You are single—maybe for a short time, maybe for a long time. You have the time for a deep spiritual journey, time like you may never have again. Why not use your sexual sabbatical as a spiritual sabbatical as well?

How far are *you* willing to go into purity? Your answer will determine the scope of your sexual revival and will definitely impact the depth of your intimacy with God. Are you where God has called you to go?

Randy told me, "Actually, I am finding it easier to see the value of sexual purity as I age. When I was in my midteens, I knew I needed to keep abstinence in mind, but it didn't carry the kind of weight that it does today. Now, at twenty-eight, I think about sexual purity all the time, because now I understand that its importance goes far beyond avoiding intercourse. It's about guarding my heart and choosing holiness in every area of my life in spite of this filthy world I live in.

"Ultimately, my sexuality is a matter of faithfulness to God, not just in obeying His commands, but also in honoring the relationship I have with Him."

Go on sabbatical, my friend. Revival is your first order of business.

where are we?

This week's reading assignment:

the introduction and chapters 1–3 in *Every Man's Battle*

Before men experience victory over sexual sin, they're hurting and confused. Why can't I win at this? *they think. As the fight wears on and the losses pile higher, we begin to doubt everything about ourselves, even our salvation. At best, we think that we're deeply flawed. At worst, evil persons. We feel very alone, since men speak little of these things.*

But we're not alone. Many men have fallen into their own sexual pits.

—from chapter 3 in *Every Man's Battle*

EVERY SINGLE MAN'S BATTLE
(Steps Along the Path to Sexual Integrity)

Experts on pornography's effects on brain chemistry recently testified at a Senate hearing about whether porn was a form of free speech that should be protected by the First Amendment or whether it was an addictive and toxic material that should be legally banned in America. Psychiatrist Jeffrey Satinover stated that it was time to quit regarding porn as just another form of expression, because it isn't. "[Porn] is a very carefully designed delivery system for evoking a tremendous flood within the brain of endogenous opioids," Satinover said. "Modern science allows us to understand that the underlying nature of an addiction to pornography is chemically nearly identical to a heroin addiction."

Dr. Mary Anne Layden, representing the Center for Cognitive Therapy at the University of Pennsylvania, explained how prurient pictures are burned into the brain's pathways. She added, "That image is in your brain forever. If that was an addictive substance, you, at any point for the rest of your life, could in a nanosecond draw it up [and get high]."

The evidence the panelists presented to the Senate that day described the overwhelming harm that pornography brings into a man's life. Still, we tend to minimize that damage from the raw visual sewage dumped into our minds and heart through our eyes. In exasperation some defenders say, *Oh, they're just exaggerating to scare everyone. Porn is just something men do to blow off stress, and they can stop anytime they want. They're not affected at all like that!*

How does porn affect you? We stated in chapter 2 that porn and masturbation inevitably inflict wounds on your sexuality. For instance, a man's eyes begin to dominate his sexuality. A boorish clamoring for his own sexual *intensity* replaces his normal desire for interpersonal *intimacy.* Controlled scientific studies have proven what many have sensed in themselves for years.

Researchers like Professors Dolf Zillman of Indiana University and Jennings Bryant of the University of Houston have found that men register a major increase in the importance of sex *without intimate attachment* after regularly viewing porn. Sound familiar? What's happening is that intimacy's transmitters get fried by porn.

Because of our discussion, it probably comes as no surprise that men who use porn become more callous to female sexuality and that married men's concern for their wives' pleasure falls off significantly. But I (Fred) know something that *will* surprise you, and that's how little porn is necessary to elicit such a dreadful, measurable change. All it takes is six one-hour weekly sessions, say the researchers.

Now look again at your life, my friend. How likely is it that porn, masturbation, and the other sensuality in your life have had no affect on your sexuality? You say none or very little? You can run to denial, but you can't hide, especially if you marry someday.

Caroline discerned the damage in her husband, Cliff, in this telling way: "About six months into our marriage, I noticed our sex life losing momentum. The frequency had dropped markedly, and while this could have easily been explained away had it been the only sign of trouble, it wasn't. We'd always been compatible—technique, frequency, timing—in every area.

"But now it was different. When we *did* make love, it felt like *Wham, bam, thank you, ma'am,* meaning Cliff got his satisfaction while I was left high and dry. I even have a journal entry that reads, 'I feel like Peg Bundy when it comes to sex. I have to nag him to do me like a chore.' It's like he stopped caring about my pleasure at all, and in retrospect, that was my first clue that porn was breaking him down."

It's important to note that the assault on healthy sexuality doesn't end at the borders of traditional pornography. The way our popular culture is set up these days—with scantily clad babes cavorting during commercials for football games, showing us their cleavage on billboards, and posing on magazine covers ranging from newsmagazines to sports—there's enough eye candy out there to keep your sexual engines running at high idle most of the time. I'm sure you've also noticed that girls and young women dress revealingly today as well, so if the porn industry vanished tomorrow, you wouldn't have to look far to take in a nice view. This lusting produces the same chemical hit to your brain as porn does, and it spins you just as easily into the same cycles of masturbation. Trust me, I know. I never did buy porn again after my wedding day, but I was just as bound in sin as I could be anyway.

You need to get serious and accept the truth. It's time to quit regarding porn as just another form of expression, and it's time to crack down on the lust of the eyes, that "carefully designed delivery system" that's been flooding your brain with opioids for years. It's time to flee sexual immorality—and time to get free.

EVERY SINGLE MAN'S TRUTH
(Your Personal Journey into God's Word)

Read and meditate upon the Bible passages below that have to do with God's holiness and His call to purity. Let the Lord remind you that He is calling you to purity because He has your best interest at heart. Also remember that He delights in you as one who is made in His image and growing into His likeness day by day.

> You have heard that it was said, "Do not commit adultery." But I tell you that anyone who looks at a woman lustfully has already committed adultery with her in his heart. (Matthew 5:27-28)

> Who will bring any charge against those whom God has chosen? It is God who justifies. Who is he that condemns? Christ Jesus, who died— more than that, who was raised to life—is at the right hand of God and is also interceding for us. Who shall separate us from the love of Christ? Shall trouble or hardship or persecution or famine or nakedness or danger or sword?… No, in all these things we are more than conquerors through him who loved us. For I am convinced that neither death nor life, neither angels nor demons, neither the present nor the future, nor any powers, neither height nor depth, nor anything else in all creation, will be able to separate us from the love of God that is in Christ Jesus our Lord. (Romans 8:33-35,37-39)

> "Come now, let us reason together,"
>   says the LORD.
> "Though your sins are like scarlet,
>   they shall be as white as snow;
> though they are red as crimson,
>   they shall be like wool." (Isaiah 1:18)

1. What do Jesus's words tell you about His deep concern for your thought life?

2. What comfort do you take in Paul's words to the Roman believers? How does this passage relate to your feelings of guilt when you've given in to lust?

3. When it comes to a believer's sin, how would you distinguish between rebellion and immaturity? What is the Father's attitude toward us as we grow—and as we stumble—in our attempts to walk in holiness with Him? (If you are a parent, think about your relationship to your children.)

4. "White as snow" is the prophet's imagery for God's holiness. To what extent do you long for holiness and purity in your life? How are Isaiah's words hopeful to you?

☑ EVERY SINGLE MAN'S CHOICE
(Questions for Personal Reflection and Examination)

📖 Pursuing sexual integrity, however, is a controversial topic.… We've been ridiculed by the world's sophisticates who find God's standard ridiculous and confining. That's fine with us, because we have a bigger concern—you.

You're in a tough position. You live in a world awash with sensual images available twenty-four hours a day in a variety of mediums: print, television, videos, the Internet—even phones. 📖

📖 After teaching on the topic of male sexual purity in Sunday school, I was approached one day by a man who said, "I always thought that since I was a man I would not be able to control my roving eyes. I didn't know it could be any other way." 📖

5. Why do you think pursuing sexual integrity is such a controversial topic, especially for singles? How realistic is this pursuit for you?

6. How aware are you of the sensual images all around you? What has been your way of dealing with—or *not* dealing with—this bombardment of sexuality on a daily basis?

7. Have you ever considered your roving eye to be uncontrollable? In the past, when have you been most likely to lose control? What has helped you to exercise control?

EVERY SINGLE MAN'S WALK
(Your Guide to Personal Application)

8. Which situations in the stories of Steve and Fred can you personally identify with most? How common do you think these kinds of situations are among the Christian men you know?

9. Think about Steve's car wreck for a moment. How much trouble have your eyes gotten you into over the years? What especially painful incident stands out to you at the moment?

10. Fred's eyes were particularly vulnerable to sensual newspaper ads. In what situations are your eyes the most vulnerable? What steps have you taken so far to avoid such situations?

11. Recall that in chapter 3 Fred speaks of the price he was paying for his sin in his relationship with God, with his family, and with his church. In which of these areas of life—or others, such as friendships and dating relationships—do you think a man's sexual sin hurts him most quickly and obviously? How is it with you?

12. In quietness, review what you have written and learned in this week's study. If further thoughts or prayer requests come to your mind and heart, you may want to write them here.

13. a. What for you was the most meaningful concept or truth in this week's study?

b. How would you talk this over with God? Write your response here as a prayer to Him.

c. What do you believe God wants you to do in response to this week's study?

👥 EVERY SINGLE MAN'S TALK
(Constructive Topics and Questions for Group Discussion)

Discussion Questions

📖 *Addictive sex is devoid of intimacy.* Sex addicts are utterly self-focused. They cannot achieve genuine intimacy because their self-obsession leaves no room for giving to others.... *Addictive sex is used to escape pain and problems.*

The escapist nature of addictive sex is often one of the clearest indicators that it is present. 📖

📖 When we're fractionally addicted, we surely experience addictive drawings, but we aren't compelled to act to salve some pain. We're compelled by the chemical high and the sexual gratification it brings.

Another way of looking at the scope of the problem is to picture a bell curve. According to our experiences, we figure around 10 percent of men have no sexual-temptation problem with their eyes and their minds. At the other end of the curve, we figure there's another 10 percent of men who are sexual addicts and have a serious problem with lust. They've been so beaten and scarred by emotional events that they simply can't overcome that sin in their lives. They need more counseling and a transforming washing by the Word. The rest of us comprise the middle 80 percent, living in various shades of gray when it comes to sexual sin. 📖

📖 "When my husband and I talked about this, he was honest," Deena conveyed, "and I was *very* angry with him. I was hurt. I felt deeply betrayed because I'd been dieting and working out to keep my weight down so that I would always look nice to him. I couldn't figure out why he still needed to look at other women."

Women told us that they struggle between pity and anger, and their feelings may ebb and flow with the tide of their husband's battle. Let us direct this advice to women reading this book: Though you know you should pray for him and fulfill him sexually, sometimes you won't want to. Talk to each other openly and honestly, then do the right thing. 📖

A. Which parts of chapters 1–3 in *Every Man's Battle* were most helpful or encouraging to you? Why?

B. How would you summarize the difference between normal sexual desire and addictive sex?

C. Do you agree that sex can be a way of trying to escape inner pain? What is your own experience with this?

D. How would you explain to another man what the authors define as *fractional addiction?*

E. To what extent do you agree or disagree with the book's contention that, for most men, our sexual sin is based on pleasure highs rather than true addiction?

F. Imagine that a single friend of yours has admitted to you, "Okay, so I use porn. A guy like me has to have *some* kind of sex life, doesn't he?" How would you respond?

G. How can indulging in visual sexual stimulation mess up a man's dating relationships? How can it make him less ready if God should call him to marriage at some time in the future?

how we got here (part A)

This week's reading assignment:

chapters 4–5 in *Every Man's Battle*

For most of us, becoming ensnared by sexual sin happened easily and naturally, like slipping off an icy log.... Perhaps you've mustered the hope that you would someday be free from sexual sin and expected to grow out of it as naturally as you grew into it—like outgrowing acne. Perhaps you waited with each birthday for your sexual impurity to clear up. It never did.

> —from chapter 4 in *Every Man's Battle*

EVERY SINGLE MAN'S BATTLE
(Steps Along the Path to Sexual Integrity)

Who draws the lines of sin in your life? If you're drawing them, then you could be in a real spot, because your standards of purity may not match God's—and you may not even know it. You may be traveling through life thinking that all is well, that you're living a pure life, yet all the while you could be running off the track, putting more distance between you and God with the passage of every day.

You'll also become discouraged in the battle when you can't seem to get completely free. You'll begin to wonder, *Perhaps there's something wrong with me!* There's nothing wrong with you. Your warped standards are still allowing enough fuel to seep in to fire your engines.

Jim, a single pastor, said that's what happened to him. "I don't understand why I'm not free yet! I've made some huge moves toward purity since reading *Every Man's Battle*—I've even gotten to the point where I'm wondering if I should be watching PG-13 movies anymore," he announced.

That point isn't far enough! Many PG-13 movies are far more naughty than nice these days. *The Hot Chick. Austin Powers: The Spy Who Shagged Me. Moulin Rouge. The Stepford Wives. The Perfect Score. Something's Gotta Give.* These are films filled with sexual innuendo, flashes of skin, and inappropriate lewdness. What's happened since PG-13 films were introduced in 1984 is that we've experienced a ratings creep where today's PG-13 movies contain significantly more sex and profanity than PG-13s did a decade ago. What was an R-rated film in the 1990s has become, in some instances, today's PG-13 fare.

How in the world did our culture sink so quickly into this sexual stew? The answer: we've dumped Scripture and lost our saltiness. "Let me tell you why you are here. You're here to be salt-seasoning that brings out the God-flavors of this earth. If you lose your saltiness, how will people taste godliness? You've lost your usefulness and will end up in the garbage" (Matthew 5:13, MSG).

That's why, when I (Fred) am drawing the lines regarding what entertainment I'll allow in *my* home, I first check out what God would allow in *His* home. Scripture lines it up for me. *Could this film be shown in heaven?* If my answer is no, there's no way I'm picking this video off the shelf at Blockbuster.

For instance, this means that blockbusters like *Forrest Gump, Braveheart,* and *Titanic* are out—their nudity breaks Ephesians 5:3 and Psalm 101:3, among many other verses.

Hold on now!

Look, I'm not being legalistic here. I don't follow God's terms this tightly because I'm under the *law* and I *must* follow. I follow this tightly because I am under *grace* and I *can* follow. It is part of my relationship with Him.

I also realize that *Braveheart* has only one nude scene (during the wedding night), and if you want to watch the rest of the movie while you turn your head away or fast-forward during that scene, I won't quarrel with you.

You are a man, as I am. Each of us will stand before God and answer for our life alone, so each of us needs to make our own decisions as we prepare for that wonderful day.

I really have only one rule: whatever pollutes is off-limits. But I'm very careful to let the Bible tell me what pollutes.

Consulting the Bible is important because if we are as desensitized to sensuality (as appears to be the case), then it's critical that we recast Scripture into the central role of our entertainment decisions. Otherwise, we'll be polluting ourselves without even realizing it.

What price are you willing to pay to get outside the cultural box and reverse your desensitization to the sensual entertainment in your life?

Mark clambered out of the box about a year ago. "I got so fed up with all of the television trash that I made a decision to stick to cable stations like the Sci Fi Channel and Animal Planet, plus some sporting events. I knew I had been seeing enough garbage to fuel my mind's sexual furnace. Once I recognized that, it only took about a month to get used to not watching those old shows, and I haven't looked back.

"It's been about a year now, and recently I picked up a season of DVDs of my favorite sci-fi show. As I was watching one of the episodes that evening, there was a rare passionate kissing scene, and as soon as it started, I felt incredibly awkward to be watching it, and I had to walk away. I wasn't numb to seeing that stuff anymore! It worked!"

See? It's all about drawing lines, so get out there and sketch up a life within God's boundaries.

EVERY SINGLE MAN'S TRUTH
(Your Personal Journey into God's Word)

Read and meditate upon the Bible passages below that deal with God's judgment and mercy—a combination powerfully demonstrated at the cross of Christ. There God's judgment upon sin mercifully freed us from having to experience its destruction. As you study, remember that God's plan is to set sinners free and then use them to teach others.

> Be imitators of God…as dearly loved children and live a life of love, just as Christ loved us and gave himself up for us as a fragrant offering and sacrifice to God.
>
> But among you there must not be even a hint of sexual immorality, or of any kind of impurity.…
>
> For you were once darkness, but now you are light in the Lord. Live as children of light (for the fruit of the light consists in all goodness, righteousness and truth) and find out what pleases the Lord. (Ephesians 5:1-3,8-10)

> It is God's will that you should be sanctified: that you should avoid sexual immorality; that each of you should learn to control his own body in a way that is holy and honorable, not in passionate lust like the heathen, who do not know God; and that in this matter no one should wrong his brother or take advantage of him. The Lord will punish men for all such sins, as we have already told you and warned you. For God did not call us to be impure, but to live a holy life. (1 Thessalonians 4:3-7)

> Have mercy on me, O God,
>   according to your unfailing love;

according to your great compassion

blot out my transgressions....

Restore to me the joy of your salvation

and grant me a willing spirit, to sustain me.

Then I will teach transgressors your ways,

and sinners will turn back to you. (Psalm 51:1,12-13)

1. What does Christ's self-sacrifice mean to you? How is it a compelling motive for holy living?

2. What does it mean for you, personally, to live as a child of the light? How can you tell when you're becoming vulnerable to the darkness?

3. How do you respond to the prospect of punishment for sin? In the past, what has been the best motivator, or encourager, to keep you from sexual impurity? What have you been doing to strengthen this motivation in your life?

4. First offer the words of Psalm 51 to God as a heartfelt prayer of your own. Then take a moment to envision how God might use you in the future to minister to another man regarding sexual purity.

☑ EVERY SINGLE MAN'S CHOICE
(Questions for Personal Reflection and Examination)

📖 That marriage doesn't eliminate sexual impurity comes as no surprise to married men, although it does for teens and young singles. Ron, a young pastor in Minnesota, said that when he challenges young men to be sexually pure, their response is, "That's easy for you to say, Pastor. You're married! You can have sex anytime you want!" Young singles believe that marriage creates a state of sexual nirvana.

If only it were so. 📖

📖 Freedom from sexual sin rarely comes through marriage or the passage of time. (The phrase "dirty old man" should tell us something about that.) So if you're tired of sexual impurity and of the mediocre, distant relationship with God that results from it, quit waiting for marriage or some hormone drop to save the day.

If you want to change, recognize that you're impure because you've diluted God's standard of sexual purity with your own. 📖

📖 God holds *you* responsible, and if you don't gain control before your wedding day, you can expect it to crop up after the honeymoon. If you're single and watching sensual R-rated movies, wedded bliss won't change this habit. If your eyes lock on passing babes, they'll still roam after you say "I do." You're masturbating now? Putting that ring on your finger won't keep your hands off yourself. 📖

5. Do you agree that marriage isn't necessarily the cure for sexual impurity? What are the practical implications of this for you if you are hoping to one day be married?

6. What irresponsible behaviors are you engaging in now that will cause problems later if you get married?

7. If you've been involved in sexual impurity, how have you experienced the distant relationship with God referred to by the authors?

8. What kinds of diluting attitudes or actions have you exhibited over the years?

EVERY SINGLE MAN'S WALK
(Your Guide to Personal Application)

Sometimes we're simply naive.... On his way [to school, Pinocchio] met some scoundrels who painted a wonderful picture of spending the day at a place called Adventure Island, a sort of amusement park just offshore.... He didn't know that at day's end all the boys would be turned into donkeys and be sold to pull carts in the coal mines....

But sometimes we choose wrong sexual standards not because we're naive, but simply because we're rebellious. We're like Lampwick, a swaggering boy who takes the lead in diverting Pinocchio to Adventure Island.... Perhaps, with a rebelliousness like Lampwick's, you know sexual immorality is wrong but you do it anyway. You love your trips to Adventure Island, despite the hidden price you pay at the end of the day.

It is holy and honorable to completely avoid sexual immorality—to repent of it, to flee from it, and to put it to death in our lives, as we live by the Spirit. We've spent enough time living like pagans in passionate lust.

9. When it comes to succumbing to temptation, would you say you are mostly naive, like Pinocchio, or mostly rebellious, like Lampwick?

10. What kinds of hidden prices have you paid at the end of a day on Adventure Island? (Take a moment to sit quietly with your regret and sadness over this. Invite the Lord's presence as you experience this pain.)

11. Prayerfully consider: what will it take for me to completely avoid sexual immorality in the weeks and years ahead? (Think about any changes in your self-image and/or God-image that may be required. Also consider what forms of accountability you may need to establish.)

12. In quietness, review what you have written and learned in this week's study. If further thoughts or prayer requests come to your mind and heart, you may want to write them here.

👥 EVERY SINGLE MAN'S TALK

(Constructive Topics and Questions for Group Discussion)

Key Highlights from the Book for Reading Aloud and Discussing

📖 In one singles Bible study group, the discussion turned to sexual purity. Many had been married before and were struggling with loneliness. When someone suggested that God expects even singles to avoid every hint of sexual immorality, one attractive young woman blurted out, "Nobody could possibly expect us to live that way!" The rest of the group heartily agreed with her, except for two who defended God's standard. 📖

📖 We aren't victims of some vast conspiracy to ensnare us sexually; we've simply chosen to mix in our own standards of sexual conduct with God's standard. Since we found God's standard too difficult, we created a mixture—something new, something comfortable, something mediocre. 📖

Discussion Questions

A. Which parts of chapter 4 in *Every Man's Battle* were most helpful or encouraging to you? Why?

B. Considering the story about the Bible study group, do you sympathize more with the majority who thought sexual purity for singles is unrealistic or with the two dissenters in the group? Why?

C. In what ways have you mixed your own sexual standards with God's? What does the resulting hodgepodge look like and feel like in your life?

D. If a man has mixed his sexuality standards with God's, what first steps can he take to get back on track? (Based upon your experience and study so far, brainstorm together about practical actions a man can take.)

E. In your own words, and in a practical way that would be helpful for single Christian men today, how would you summarize God's standards for sexual purity?

Note: If you're following a twelve-week track,
save the rest of this lesson for the following week.
If you're on the eight-week track, then keep going.

☑ EVERY SINGLE MAN'S CHOICE
(Questions for Personal Reflection and Examination)

📖 Is it profitable for Christians to stop short at the middle ground of excellence where costs are low, balanced somewhere between paganism and obedience? Not at all! While in business it's profitable to *seem* perfect, in the spiritual realm it's merely *comfortable* to seem perfect....

Excellence is a *mixed* standard, while obedience is a *fixed* standard. We want to shoot for the fixed standard. 📖

📖 If we don't kill every hint of immorality, we'll be captured by our tendency as males to draw sexual gratification and chemical highs through our eyes.… But we can't deal with our maleness until we first reject our right to mix standards. As we ask "How holy can I be?" we must pray and commit to a new relationship with God, fully aligned with His call to obedience. 📖

13. How would you explain the difference between the pursuit of excellence and the pursuit of perfection (through obedience)?

14. Do you believe you have a right, at least sometimes, to mix your own standards with God's?

15. Consider the difference in attitude reflected in these two personal questions: *How far can I go and still be called a Christian? How holy can I be?* How would these attitudes likely manifest themselves in an unmarried man's actions?

👟 EVERY SINGLE MAN'S WALK
(Your Guide to Personal Application)

📖 God is your Father and expects obedience. Having given you the Holy Spirit as your power source, He believes His command should be enough for you....

Trouble is, we aren't in search of obedience. We're in search of mere excellence, and His command is *not* enough. We push back, responding, "*Why* should I eliminate every hint? That's too hard!" 📖

📖 What's your Christian life costing you?

It costs *something* to learn about Christ. It costs *a lot* to live like Christ. It costs something to join a few thousand men at a conference to sing praises to God and learn how we should live; it costs a lot to come home and remain committed to the changes you said you'd make in your life....

It costs a lot to control your eyes and mind daily. 📖

16. How would you respond to someone who says, "Why should I eliminate every hint of sexual impurity?"

17. Think through some of the impure temptations and/or practices you've been able to eliminate from your life so far. What hints still remain?

18. Realistically, what is it costing you these days to be a Christian? Try making a list of some of your spiritual price tags. What insight does this list offer?

19. What will likely be the next challenge for you, just over the horizon, when it comes to controlling your eyes and mind? What preparations have you made in order to be ready for the onslaught of temptation?

20. a. What for you was the most meaningful concept or truth in this week's study?

    b. How would you talk this over with God? Write your response here as a prayer to Him.

c. What do you believe God wants you to do in response to this week's study?

👥 EVERY SINGLE MAN'S TALK
(More Topics and Questions for Group Discussion)

Key Highlights from the Book for Reading Aloud and Discussing

📖 I…organized an intercessors' group during our church's Wednesday night services, simply opening a room for ninety minutes of intercession for our congregation. The first night, a half-dozen people came to the door and asked, "Is this the room where they're teaching about intercession?"

"No, we won't be *teaching* about intercession," I answered. "We're going to *be* interceding." Each person turned away to leave. It feels good to learn about intercession, but it's a costly thing to do. The same can be said about purity. 📖

📖 Sexual impurity has become rampant in the church because we've ignored the costly work of obedience to God's standards as individuals, asking too often, "How far can I go and still be called a Christian?" We've crafted an image and may even *seem* sexually pure while permitting our eyes to play freely when no one is around, avoiding the hard work of *being* sexually pure. 📖

Discussion Questions

F. Which parts of chapter 5 in *Every Man's Battle* were most helpful or encouraging to you? Why?

G. What was the last lie you told (about anything)? How do single men tend to modify the truth in their approach to sexual purity?

H. Why is it so much easier to learn about prayer than to pray? to learn about purity than to practice purity? What are some of the highest costs involved?

I. Look together at the story of King Josiah in 2 Chronicles 34. Read aloud verse 8 and verses 14-33. How do you see Josiah's example in this passage as a model of obedience? What else is Josiah's example here a model of?

J. When are your eyes most likely to play freely? Talk together about actions or attitudes that help you control your eyes. (Be willing to share what works for you.)

K. Are God's standards on sexuality for single people starting to look more appealing to you? more attainable? Why or why not?

how we got here (part B)

This week's reading assignment:

chapters 6–7 in *Every Man's Battle*

You stand before an important battle. You've decided that the slavery of sexual sin isn't worth your love of sexual sin. You're committed to removing every hint of it. But how? Your maleness looms as your own worse enemy.

You got into this mess by being male; you'll get out by being a man.

—from chapter 7 in *Every Man's Battle*

EVERY SINGLE MAN'S BATTLE
(Steps Along the Path to Sexual Integrity)

One wintry Saturday morning a few years ago, I (Fred) retreated to the family basement and laid a full-court press on my Dell laptop to meet a writing deadline. Upstairs, my wife, Brenda, tried to cope with four kids who had to stay indoors because of blustery Iowa winds and a steel gray sky. With everyone dancing on one another's nerves, Brenda embarked on a dependable course of action: when the going gets tough, the tough go shopping.

Brenda shuttled our gang over to the mall, and upon their return, I heard them burst through the door amid peels of laughter with large, lumpy bags stuffed with plunder clunking to the floor. As our children scattered across the house to their various pursuits, a satisfied peace settled over the house—until my youngest son, Michael, snuck up behind Brenda and put his arms around her for a hug.

Turning around with a smile, she offered him her soft arms only to discover a pair of searching eyes leveled upon hers. "Mom, how do you get pictures of women in their underwear out of your head?" he implored.

Did I really hear that? she wondered, knowing that Michael was just eleven years old and innocent for his age.

She regained her equilibrium, and like any battle-tested mom, she didn't miss a beat. "I think I hear your dad calling you," she replied.

He turned around and was about to scamper down the stairs to look for me when she asked, "Michael, before you go, exactly what kind of pictures are you talking about?"

"Remember when we walked to the food court for lunch today?

"Sure."

"Well, we walked past that secret store, and after I looked up into the store window, I haven't been able to get those pictures out of my head all day."

Suddenly everything clicked for Brenda—and for me when Michael told me what had happened. That "secret store" was none other than Victoria's Secret, and I needn't explain to you what he saw in that window display that afternoon. Perhaps consciously for the first time, Michael experienced the ability of male eyes to lock in sensual images with only a glance.

Don't miss an important point here. Michael was only eleven—he wouldn't have known a girl from a bale of hay, I assure you! He wasn't lusting, and he wasn't looking for something racy to make his day. He was simply being male, one little guy minding his own business who happened to glance in a certain direction at a certain time. Yet it still happened—his eyes *still* locked and loaded that image into his brain.

As we said in *Every Man's Battle,* this is the one big reason for the prevalence of sexual sin among us guys, even apart from our tendency to stop short of God's standards. We get there naturally—simply by being male.

Your eyes will work the way they were designed to. Your job is to train them to move in step with your faith and to face that difficult assignment of integrating your sexuality with the emotional, spiritual, and relational person you want to be.

Now here's the problem. Because decades' worth of 50 percent divorce rates have cut off countless fathers from their sons, and because a Sexual Code of Silence prevents any *serious* discussion about sex from taking place with other men, many of us have the tendency to see our sexuality as something shamefully separate from ourselves, even into our later years. Don't go there at all.

Shame has no part in this equation. After all, as you've seen in Michael's story, the ability of the male eyes and mind to draw sexual gratification from the world is simply a fact of life for us. With all this foreplay of the eyes going on, and little guidance on what to do with these feelings as you moved through your teens and twenties, the warped results you've seen in yourself are understandable. There's nothing defective in you per se, so why be ashamed? You're just a normal guy who needs to learn how to manage his sex drive. That's part of becoming a man for any guy.

Sure, the battle's landscape has changed dramatically with the Internet and MTV, and we're largely getting blasted off the spiritual battlefield. Today's blitzkrieg of visual stimulation has our senses on high alert at all times. But since our nature sets us up to fail in this sexually charged culture—unless someone taught us early how to control our eyes, mind, and passions—there's no sense in pounding ourselves over the head with shame over this. It comes with the territory.

You are male, so you have a visual fight on your hands. Sooner or later you must engage that battle.

It's time to step up like a man and deal with it.

📖 EVERY SINGLE MAN'S TRUTH
(Your Personal Journey into God's Word)

As you begin this study, ask for the Holy Spirit's help in hearing and obeying His personal words for you. Read and meditate upon the Bible passages below that have to do with God's call to sexual faithfulness. As you read realize that God is not calling you to anything that's foreign to Himself. The Scriptures proclaim over and over again the Lord's utter faithfulness…to *you!*

> These commands are a lamp,
>   this teaching is a light,
> and the corrections of discipline
>   are the way to life,
> keeping you from the immoral woman,
>   from the smooth tongue of the wayward wife.
> Do not lust in your heart after her beauty
>   or let her captivate you with her eyes,
> for the prostitute reduces you to a loaf of bread,
>   and the adulteress preys upon your very life.
> Can a man scoop fire into his lap
>   without his clothes being burned?
> Can a man walk on hot coals
>   without his feet being scorched?…
> But a man who commits adultery lacks judgment;
>   whoever does so destroys himself. (Proverbs 6:23-28,32)

Among you there must not be even a hint of sexual immorality, or of any kind of impurity…because these are improper for God's holy people. (Ephesians 5:3)

[Treat] younger women as sisters, with absolute purity. (1 Timothy 5:2)

> He will cover you with his feathers,
>> and under his wings you will find refuge;
>> his faithfulness will be your shield and rampart. (Psalm 91:4)

1. What are some of the horrible consequences of lust, fornication, and adultery? How does a man destroy himself in the arms of a woman who is not his wife?

2. What kinds of changes would not even permitting a *hint* of sexual immorality and treating women with *absolute* purity require in your life?

3. When you think of God's faithfulness to you, what events or circumstances of the past spring to mind? (Spend some moments in thankfulness and praise.)

4. How does it feel to know that God's love is like the warm and close protection that a hen offers its young? How can God's faithfulness act as a "shield and rampart" in your life?

5. How easy or difficult is it for you, after you have fallen to temptation, to immediately move back under God's wings? Why?

☑ EVERY SINGLE MAN'S CHOICE

(Questions for Personal Reflection and Examination)

📖 *For males, impurity of the eyes is sexual foreplay.*

That's right. Just like stroking an inner thigh or rubbing a breast. Because foreplay is any sexual action that naturally takes us down the road to intercourse. Foreplay ignites passions, rocketing us by stages until we go all the way....

No doubt about it: Visual sexual gratification is a form of sex for men. As males we draw sexual gratification and chemical highs through our eyes.

📖 In a newsletter, author and speaker Dr. Gary Rosberg told of seeing a pair of hands that reminded him of the hands of his father, who had gone on to heaven. Gary continued to reminisce about what his father's hands meant to him. Then he shifted his thoughts to the hands of Jesus, noting this simple truth: "They were hands that never touched a woman with dishonor." 📖

6. Have you ever before considered the dangers of visual foreplay? What is your reaction to the authors' statements about it?

7. What role is visual sexual gratification playing in your life these days? What is your level of awareness of it?

8. Think about the reputation of Jesus's hands for a moment. Then consider: what legacy will your hands leave behind?

9. Read Galatians 6:7-8. How have you seen the truth of this principle in your own life?

EVERY SINGLE MAN'S WALK

(Your Guide to Personal Application)

I (Fred) remember the moment…when it all broke loose. I'd failed God with my eyes for the thirty-millionth time. My heart churned in guilt, pain, and sorrow. Driving down Merle Hay Road, I suddenly gripped the wheel and through clenched teeth, I yelled out: "That's it! I'm through with this! I'm making a covenant with my eyes. I don't care what it takes, and I don't care if I die trying. It stops here. It stops *here!*"

I made that covenant and built it brick by brick…. My breakthrough:

- I made a clear decision.
- I decided once and for all to make a change….

I wasn't fully convinced I could trust myself even then, but I'd finally and truly engaged the battle. Through my covenant with my eyes, all my mental and spiritual resources were now leveled upon a single target: my impurity.

With that covenant I had also chosen manhood, to rise above my natural male tendencies. That was a huge step for me.

Was God proud of Job? You bet!… In Job 31:1, we see Job making this startling revelation: "I made a covenant with my eyes not to look lustfully at a girl."

A covenant with his eyes! You mean he made a promise with his eyes to not gaze upon a young woman? It's not possible! It can't be true!

Yet Job was successful; otherwise, he wouldn't have made this promise: "If my heart has been enticed by a woman, or if I have lurked at my neighbor's door, then may my wife grind another man's grain, and may other men sleep with her" (31:9).

10. Fred had failed "thirty million" times. How many times has it been for you? Do you believe it will take a crisis like Fred's to bring you to a place of choosing covenant making? Why or why not?

11. Have you ever sensed that the grace of God was the only way out of your cycle of failed willpower? How did you respond?

12. What does it mean for you to rest in God's saving grace? How will you know when you are ready to make that your standard response during the toughest temptations?

13. If you were to make a covenant with your eyes right now, how would you write it? Jot your statement here:

14. In quietness, review what you have written and learned in this week's study. If further thoughts or prayer requests come to your mind and heart, you may want to write them here.

15. a. What for you was the most meaningful concept or truth in this week's study?

    b. How would you talk this over with God? Write your response here as a prayer to Him.

    c. What do you believe God wants you to do in response to this week's study?

◎◎ EVERY SINGLE MAN'S TALK
(Constructive Topics and Questions for Group Discussion)

Key Highlights from the Book for Reading Aloud and Discussing

📖 Author George Gilder in *Sexual Suicide* reported that men commit more than 90 percent of major crimes of violence, 100 percent of the rapes, and 95 percent of the burglaries. Men comprise 94 percent of our drunken drivers, 70 percent of suicides, 91 percent of offenders against family and children. Most often, the chief perpetrators are single men.

Our maleness brings a natural, uniquely male form of rebelliousness. This natural tendency gives us the arrogance needed to stop short of God's standards. As men, we'll often choose sin simply because we like our own way. 📖

📖 When it comes down to it, God's definition of real manhood is pretty simple: It means hearing His Word and *doing it.* That's God's *only* definition of manhood—a doer of the Word. And God's definition of a sissy is someone who hears the Word of God and *doesn't* do it. 📖

Discussion Questions

A. Which parts of chapters 6 and 7 in *Every Man's Battle* were most helpful or encouraging to you? Why?

B. "Males are rebellious by nature." Obviously this trait is not a gift from God but a result of our sin nature as fallen human beings. Think about other male traits. To what degree is each one a gift from God? To what degree is each one a result of our sin nature?

C. How would you describe the difference between maleness and manhood?

D. In our culture, what are the stereotypes about the lifestyle of a single man? How do these stereotypes differ from biblical manhood as it applies to single men?

E. Do you totally buy into the conclusion that a real man is one who is a doer of the Word of God? Why or why not?

F. How important is the fellowship of other Christian men when it comes to your ability to be a doer of the Word? What are the opportunities for forming accountability relationships within your group? Talk about it.

choosing victory (part A)

This week's reading assignment:

chapter 8 in *Every Man's Battle*

When you talk to courageous…World War II veterans…they say they don't feel like heroes. They simply had a job to do. When the landing-craft ramps fell open, they swallowed hard and said, "It's time." Time to fight.

In your struggle with sexual impurity, isn't it time? Sure, fighting back will be hard.

Your life…[is] under a withering barrage of machine-gun sexuality that rakes the landscape mercilessly. Right now you're in a landing craft, inching closer to shore and a showdown. God has given you the weapons and trained you for battle.

You can't stay in the landing craft forever.

—from chapter 8 in *Every Man's Battle*

EVERY SINGLE MAN'S BATTLE
(Steps Along the Path to Sexual Integrity)

You've had the power to win the battle for purity from the day you were saved. Granted, you may be feeling like you have *no* power right now. I (Fred) have worn those same chains, so I know exactly how you feel. But now that I've thrown off those chains, I can see clearly that whether you sense that power is inside you or not, it's there just the same and is able to work on your behalf.

I sure wasn't aware that God's power had arrived the night I asked Him into my life. It all began one forlorn evening in my office in Palo Alto, California, when I prayed, "God, I'm ready to work with You, if You're ready to work with me."

I didn't feel anything at the time. I simply stood up, wiped away my tears, and headed out to my car to head home for the evening. I didn't know for sure what I had done or even whether I was saved, but that didn't matter. God began working in my life, and the power was inside me just the same.

A few weeks later I headed back to my home state to start a new job. After I settled into an apartment in Ankeny, Iowa, my nights were monotonous and long. A man accustomed to juggling four girlfriends wasn't used to having his nights free!

In no time, thoughts of someone new—Janet—swirled in my imagination. She was an old friend from high school, and I'd been enamored with her for years. Back then I'd been too busy with football to start a relationship with Janet, but I'd often dreamed of sleeping with her.

I soon tracked her down and—what luck! She was still single and living in Omaha, a couple of hours away. I called her and, after some cheerful banter, she invited me to meet her at her favorite dance bar. Need I say more? After closing time, we found ourselves alone in her apartment. One thing led to another, and we slipped out of our clothes and into her bed. We began kissing, but a strange thing happened: I couldn't get an erection! Now *that* had never happened before. Deeply humiliated, and with my head spinning, I slunk out to the parking lot and into my car.

Then I clearly heard the Holy Spirit whisper into my heart, "By the way, I did that to you. I know it hurt you, but this practice can't be tolerated anymore in your life. You are Christ's now, and He loves you." He didn't have to say it twice—on the spot I recommitted myself to staying pure.

But if we all have this great power inside us, why aren't we all pure?

Great question! Sadly, there's an easy answer: we can say no to that new life in us and stop its work in our life. If you're saying, "Huh?" then let me demonstrate this with the following story.

If the power of the new life of Christ had ever been evident in anyone, it was in Tim, a man who cornered me after I spoke one night in Long Island, New York. "I'm thankful for your practical message tonight," he said as he pulled me aside. "My story really backs you up."

"I'd love to hear about it," I said, intrigued.

"Though I have a wonderful wife who really takes care of me in bed, I've always had eyes for women and Internet porn, which led to a problem with masturbation for years. I cried and prayed long and hard for God to deliver me. One night, as I slept, I believe He did."

"Really?"

"Yes, really. I had a dream where I was standing cold and lonely in a vast dark room, frightened and unable to get out. Suddenly, a spotlight shone straight down on me from above, and a pure white raiment floated down and settled over me, covering me in His grace.

"The next day I noticed that the pull toward porn had vanished. The desire was simply gone. I praised God all day, and I continued praising Him as the days and weeks passed without making any late-night visits to the computer."

"Wow, that's great!" I exclaimed. "What a story!"

"Oh, but wait. Unfortunately and sadly, that's not the end. While God had delivered me miraculously, I never really dealt with my character or my looking-around habits. Last summer I was still staring long at the babes walking by with their breasts half hanging out. Before long, one girl with particularly large breasts got me pretty excited, which tripped a memory of someone who looked exactly like her at some porn site on the Internet. The next time I got online, I thought, *It wouldn't hurt to take a quick peek. I'm delivered, after all. It can't hurt me.*"

I knew what was coming.

"Well, that one peek led to many more looks over the next few weeks, and today I'm as stuck as I ever was."

The power of God is awesome and is ever present in you, right from the beginning of your Christian life. But as we've seen in Tim's story, even if God were to multiply that power and miraculously free you in a moment of time, you'd still have to learn to flee, or you could fall right back into your addiction. Like the filth from a broken sewage pipe, this stuff will seep into your mind and keep you from experiencing the victory you'd love to enjoy.

EVERY SINGLE MAN'S TRUTH
(Your Personal Journey into God's Word)

As you begin this study, read and meditate upon the Bible passages below that have to do with your identity and power in Christ. Remember that Christ has already fought the battle against sin on your behalf—and won. Now it is time to live in that victory every day.

> Grace and peace be yours in abundance through the knowledge of God and of Jesus our Lord.
>
> His divine power has given us everything we need for life and godliness through our knowledge of him who called us by his own glory and goodness. Through these he has given us his very great and precious promises, so that through them you may participate in the divine nature and escape the corruption in the world caused by evil desires. (2 Peter 1:2-4)

> If we died with Christ, we believe that we will also live with him. For we know that since Christ was raised from the dead, he cannot die again; death no longer has mastery over him. The death he died, he died to sin once for all; but the life he lives, he lives to God.
>
> In the same way, count yourselves dead to sin but alive to God in Christ Jesus. Therefore do not let sin reign in your mortal body so that you obey its evil desires. Do not offer the parts of your body to sin, as instru-

ments of wickedness, but rather offer yourselves to God, as those who have been brought from death to life; and offer the parts of your body to him as instruments of righteousness. For sin shall not be your master, because you are not under law, but under grace.…

You have been set free from sin and have become slaves to righteousness. (Romans 6:8-14,18)

1. According to Peter, what exactly has God given you? What is the source of your ability to "participate in the divine nature"? When have you most powerfully sensed the glory and goodness of Jesus in your life?

2. If we have everything we need for godliness, what is holding us back from lifelong sexual purity? (Think about what it means to count yourself dead to sin.)

3. In the heat of sexual temptation, what will it mean for you to, as Paul says, *not* "offer…your body to sin"? What will offering yourself to God require at that point? (Give some thought to the role your willpower can play—and *can't* play—at this point in the battle.)

4. Have you ever known someone who was a slave to righteousness? What can you learn from him or her?

☑ EVERY SINGLE MAN'S CHOICE
(Questions for Personal Reflection and Examination)

📖 I was angry. I wanted to win right away and to win decisively—not somewhere down the road where age might bring victory through the back door. I wanted to win when the battle was hottest.

You should too. If you don't win now, you'll never know whether you're truly a man of God. 📖

📖 We've known those who have failed in their battle for sexual purity, and we know some who have won. The difference? Those who won hated their impurity. They were going to war and were going to win—or die trying. Every resource was leveled upon the foe.

There will be no victory in this area of your life until you choose manhood with all your might. 📖

5. How angry are you about the battle? On a scale of one to ten, how convinced are you that God's will is for you to win the battle and be sexually pure?

6. On a scale of one to ten, to what extent would you say that you truly hate the sin of sexual impurity in any form?

7. On a scale of one to ten, to what extent would you say you truly expect to win the battle for sexual purity? What are your reasons for picking this score?

👟 Every Single Man's Walk

(Your Guide to Personal Application)

📖 Listen to the…words spoken by preacher Steve Hill, who was addressing escape from addiction to drugs and alcohol as well as from sexual sin: "There's no temptation that is uncommon to man. God will send you a way of escape, but you've got to be willing to take that way of escape, friend." 📖

📖 Admit it: You love your sexual highs, but slavery engulfs you. Is the love worth the loathing?…

Look in the mirror. Are you proud of your sexual fantasizing? Or do you feel degraded after viewing lingerie ads or sex scenes in films?

Sexually speaking, you have a low-grade sexual fever. It doesn't disable you, but you aren't healthy either. You can sort of function normally, but you can't really push hard. Basically, you just get by. And if this fever doesn't break, you'll never fully function as a Christian. Like the prodigal, you need to come to your senses and make a decision. 📖

8. What is your strongest motivation for achieving and maintaining sexual purity?

9. Recall some of the times when you gave in to sexual temptation. Was there always a "way of escape" open to you? In a particular instance, what do you think kept you from taking the escape route?

10. Answer Steve and Fred's question as honestly as you can: "Is the love worth the loathing?" (Suggestion: for a few minutes, turn your awareness to Christ's abiding presence. Just you and Jesus—sit quietly together with your response.)

11. Read Romans 12:1-2. Imagine completely giving up sexual fantasy in your life. How much grief would that bring you? Are you ready to experience that pain as an act of sacrificial worship?

12. In quietness, review what you have written and learned in this week's study. If further thoughts or prayer requests come to your mind and heart, you may want to write them here.

13. a. What for you was the most meaningful concept or truth in this week's study?

    b. How would you talk this over with God? Write your response here as a prayer to Him.

c. What do you believe God wants you to do in response to this week's study?

👥 EVERY SINGLE MAN'S TALK
(Constructive Topics and Questions for Group Discussion)

Key Highlights from the Book for Reading Aloud and Discussing

📖 Sexual impurity isn't like a tumor growing out of control inside us. We treat it that way when our prayers focus on *deliverance,* as we plead for someone to come remove it. Actually, sexual impurity is a series of bad decisions on our part—a result of immature character—and deliverance won't deliver you into instant maturity. Character work needs to be done.

Holiness is not some nebulous thing. It's a series of right choices.... You'll be holy when you choose not to sin. You're already free from the *power* of sexual immorality; you are not yet free from the *habit* of sexual immorality, until you choose to be. 📖

📖 Regarding sexual purity, God knows the provision He's made for us. We aren't short on power or authority, but what we lack is *urgency.* We must choose to be strong and courageous to walk into purity. In the millisecond it takes to make that choice, the Holy Spirit will start guiding you and walking through the struggle with you. 📖

Discussion Questions

A. Which parts of chapter 8 in *Every Man's Battle* were most helpful or encouraging to you? Why?

B. Consider the out-of-control tumor analogy. Why do we tend to think of sexual impurity as a disease that attacks us? How is this a cop-out?

C. What is wrong with praying for deliverance year after year?

D. Describe as clearly and concisely as you can the provision God has made for us.

E. Talk in practical terms about what choosing means to you.

F. What are some other tough choices you have made in the past? What motivated you to make those choices? What can you learn from those experiences to help you make the choice to live a holy life in the area of your sexuality?

G. Take a few moments as a group to reflect silently on these questions as they apply and relate to you. How long are you going to stay sexually impure? How long will you behave immorally with a girlfriend? How long will you put off becoming the kind of man your future wife can respect and trust?

choosing victory (part B)

This week's reading assignment:

chapters 9–10 in *Every Man's Battle*

Okay, so you've decided it's time to fight. And you realize that your battle for sexual purity will cost you something. It will require sacrifice, intensity, and honor.

But let's get something else in clear view: What can you expect to gain *by choosing manhood and the purity that goes with it?*

By winning this war, your life will be blessed in tremendous ways. Your victory will recover what was lost through sin.

—from chapter 9 in *Every Man's Battle*

Every Single Man's Battle
(Steps Along the Path to Sexual Integrity)

In 1 Thessalonians 4:4, God clearly expressed His will for you: "Each of you should learn to control his own body in a way that is holy and honorable." God wants you to control your life by using *His* weapons. God is a strong God, and He wants you to be a strong man. So, what are you going to do with the sexual pressure you some-times feel? First of all, once you get your eyes and mind under control, the sexual pressure will drop off dramatically. As singles we bring most of the sexual pressure onto ourselves through visual stimulation and mental fantasy.

You may be thinking, *Even so, what about that male seventy-two-hour cycle of sperm production you talk about in* Every Man's Battle?

While there's still some natural physical pressure for release from time to time, it normally weakens in singles. The regular sexual release in marriage seems to ramp up the pressure from this cycle in married men. As for singles, we've seen that without this regular sexual release, the cycle of desire often goes to sleep or "dries up."

Thad is twice divorced and forty-three years old. "For a single man, there are no acceptable sexual outlets," he said, "but I've found that if I keep the right perspectives and live cleanly, the pressure dissipates.

"But it *is* difficult to abstain from sexual activity at times, especially in a culture where I am surrounded by sexual images and opportunities. This is where emotion-ally, intellectually, and spiritually intimate relationships with other men can provide the support I need to be faithful in my relationship with God. Ultimately, my sexual-ity is a matter of faithfulness to God—not just obeying His commands but also hon-oring my relationship with Him."

God has helped us honor our relationships with Him by providing a couple of built-in relief valves. The first—nocturnal emissions—was mentioned in *Every Man's Battle,* and these emissions are there to release the buildup of sperm. But whether this valve kicks in to help you or not, God has built in a second natural mechanism for all of us, and it's this: excess sperm is simply dumped into the bladder and passed with the urine. The important thing to know is that once you've eliminated the sexual pressure that comes from sexual impurity, these mechanisms are capable of taking care of any problem arising from ongoing sperm production.

Rob, a never-married thirty-year-old, told us about his situation: "I never actually put forth a sincere effort toward purity until the past few months, and I haven't masturbated for a while. Has it been easy? Yes, surprisingly so. But at the same time, I've been guarding my eyes and my mind passionately. I don't think I could go without some sort of release if I wasn't guarding myself from the temptation."

Many singles think God's unfair to ask us to duke it out at all. As the frustration rises, they snap, "God is so unfair to make us sexual and then to forbid sex altogether!" It can sure look that way from our perspective as single men—a perspective limited mainly to our concern with how *His* ways intensify *our* battle for sexual purity.

But God's ways are so much higher than your ways that He's often got your back even while you're frowning in frustration. To you, He's unfair, unconcerned about what you *want*—a sweet sexual outlet, an easy way out of the battle. But that's only because He's so concerned about what you *need*—protection from self-inflicted damage to your sexual hard drive that comes from porn and masturbation. He loves you, so He can't offer sex with yourself as an outlet.

God can't offer sex with others either. He loves them, too! As the Creator, He understands the purposes of sex far too well to offer up women, no matter how willing or available, as your sexual outlet. For one thing, He made sex to uniquely cement you to a woman's soul so as to create a safe, unbroken home for raising godly offspring.

Ah, but He *also* knows that this sexual glue bonds to any surface, and premarital sexual relationships can cement you into wrong, unhealthy relationships as easily as that right one in marriage. So when you consider that premarital sex also short-circuits the natural development of the very relationships that you are blindly gluing in place, perhaps you ought to thank Him for being so "unfair" to you.

Once we get *that* perspective, it becomes easier to see the point of waiting on sex. William is twice divorced, forty-eight, and single, and he's finally getting the hang of God's perspectives on sex. "The older I get, the more clearly I see the beauty of sexual purity and necessity for relational intimacy to progress in a natural way without the physical intimacy."

That's the road we want to be traveling on, guys.

📖 EVERY SINGLE MAN'S TRUTH
(Your Personal Journey into God's Word)

The Bible passages below continue with the theme of our identity and power in Christ. As you consider their message, ask the Holy Spirit to lead you into specific, practical applications for your daily life.

> Do you not know that your bodies are members of Christ himself? Shall I then take the members of Christ and unite them with a prostitute? Never! Do you not know that he who unites himself with a prostitute is one with her in body? For it is said, "The two will become one flesh." But he who unites himself with the Lord is one with him in spirit.
>
> Flee from sexual immorality. All other sins a man commits are outside his body, but he who sins sexually sins against his own body. (1 Corinthians 6:15-18)

> We take captive every thought to make it obedient to Christ. (2 Corinthians 10:5)

> I keep asking that the God of our Lord Jesus Christ, the glorious Father, may give you the Spirit of wisdom and revelation, so that you may know him better. I pray also that the eyes of your heart may be enlightened in order that you may know the hope to which he has called you, the riches of his glorious inheritance in the saints, and his incomparably great power for us who believe. That power is like the working of his mighty strength, which he exerted in Christ when he raised him from the dead and seated him at his right hand in the heavenly realms, far above all rule and authority, power and dominion, and every title that can be given, not only in the present age but also in the one to come. (Ephesians 1:17-21)

1. According to 1 Corinthians 6, what is a major implication of being "in Christ"? Have you ever thought of your body as being a part of Christ? What does this mean to you?

2. When are your thoughts typically most captive to Christ? When are they most likely to roam free and get you into trouble?

3. Paul wanted believers to know Jesus better. How can knowing Him well help us stay sexually pure? How can knowing Him better, day by day, bring power into our lives? (Think about some practical applications to your own battle.)

☑ EVERY SINGLE MAN'S CHOICE
(Questions for Personal Reflection and Examination)

📖 Because of sin, I (Fred) hadn't been able to look at myself in a mirror for years. While I knew God loved me unconditionally, I also knew He didn't unconditionally approve of my behavior. Consequently, I couldn't look God in the eye.

Once I heard a pastor preach, "When Jesus knocks, He wants freedom to enter every room in your house. In every part of your life, He wants to be welcome and comfortable. Is He locked out of any room in your house?" 📖

📖 I (Fred) was a prodigal eating old cobs of corn left in a pigsty. To restore my relationship with my Father, I had to get up out of the mud and start walking home. I didn't have to clean myself up first, but I did have to make that first step. On the road ahead, the Father would be waiting with a ring, a robe, shoes, and everything else an honored son was meant to have. But first I had to come to my senses, as I did that day on Merle Hay Road when I took my first step toward home—toward purity—by making that covenant with my eyes. 📖

4. Can you look at yourself in the mirror these days? Can you look God in the eye? Why or why not?

5. Make a list of the rooms in your inner house where Jesus is welcome and unwelcome. What keeps certain rooms off-limits to Him, even though He already knows what's there? (Suggestion: spend some moments right now letting Jesus into the ugliest rooms. Tell Him of the longing, desire, pain, and so on that have helped you furnish those rooms over the years. This is an opportunity to open your whole heart to Him.)

6. If you see some aspects of the prodigal son within you, where are you in your journey? Are you still heading for adventure in the big, wide world? suffering loss and desperation? on your way back home?

EVERY SINGLE MAN'S WALK
(Your Guide to Personal Application)

One of the things I (Steve) brought into my marriage with Sandy was a secret compartment I'd guarded for years. Inside it was a girlfriend from much earlier in my life, the first true love I really had.... I considered this secret compartment to be mine forever, a private place out of which I could draw fond old memories.

Sin can affect families for generations, as it did in mine. I came from a family in which the men loved sex and pornography and ditched their wives or were caught up in affairs....

My sixteen-year-old son, Jasen, is now a handsome, strapping, six-foot adolescent with an easy smile and friendly ways. Not long ago Jasen was with friends who had some pornography. He walked away. *My son walked away.* You don't understand what that means to me!

7. To what extent can you relate to Steve's secret compartment? Do you have any compartments labeled Old Girlfriends or Pornography or Favorite Web Sites? What practical steps can you take—today—to begin forsaking these private, secret compartments?

8. How have you been affected by the sins of your father and other males in your family? If you have children (or hope to have children one day), how do you think your secret sins of impurity might affect them?

9. Be Fred for a moment. How do you feel after discovering that Jasen walked away from pornography? Would your son (or any child who looks to your example, such as a nephew or a teen you teach in Sunday school) walk away?

10. As you think of attaining the sexual purity that is God's will for you, how do you envision your relationship with God in the near future? your relationship with your future wife and children? your church ministry in the near future and long term?

11. In quietness, review what you have written and learned in this week's study. If further thoughts or prayer requests come to your mind and heart, you may want to write them here.

EVERY SINGLE MAN'S TALK
(Constructive Topics and Questions for Group Discussion)

Key Highlights from the Book for Reading Aloud and Discussing

Along with inner peace comes an outer peace that affects your daily life. In an earlier chapter I mentioned a businessman named Wally and his dread of hotels. Wally can now check into a hotel at night, enjoy a meal at the coffee shop, go back to his room, shower, turn out the lights, and fall asleep. "I no longer fear hotel rooms in the slightest," he says. "Sensual things don't dominate my day as they once could."

Trust is important in the body of Christ. In 1 Corinthians 6:15-20, Paul says that not only does a sexually immoral man sin against his own body, but he also sins against the body of Christ and his friends within the body.

Our friends trust us to be pure; a failure would crush their spirits as well as our own. We must be trustworthy. 📖

📖 When your son questions what he should watch, what he should do with the pornography other boys show him, or what he should do when that cute girl gets him alone and starts unbuttoning her blouse, will anyone be speaking against it? It won't be his friends. Even his *church* buddies will tell him to go for it. *Your* voice had better be loud and crystal clear because it will probably be the only one whispering, "Flee immorality, son." Your *example* must be the argument opposing temptation. 📖

Discussion Questions

A. Which parts of chapter 9 in *Every Man's Battle* were most helpful or encouraging to you? Why?

B. Talk about Wally and the change that occurred in his life. In your opinion, how realistic is it to think that any man could come to the point of not being tempted by the X-rated cable channels in a motel room?

C. Talk together about the trust levels in your group in light of the middle quotation above. Discuss some ways you can maintain trust with one another in the area of sexual purity.

D. Look at the third quotation above. Sit for a while in silence as each man does a personal check within his heart. Then spend some time praying for one another's children (if you have them) and/or for the young men in your church or community.

Note: If you're following a twelve-week track,
save the rest of this lesson for the following week.
If you're on the eight-week track, then keep going.

☑ EVERY SINGLE MAN'S CHOICE
(Questions for Personal Reflection and Examination)

📖 Satan's greatest weapon against you is…deception. He knows Jesus has already purchased your freedom. He also knows that once you see the simplicity of this battle, you'll win in short order, so he deceives and confuses. He tricks you into thinking you're a helpless victim, someone who'll need years of group therapy. 📖

📖 Your goal is sexual purity. Here's a good working definition of it—good because of its simplicity:

You are sexually pure when no sexual gratification comes from anyone or anything but your wife.

Purity means stopping sexual gratification that comes to us from outside our marriage. 📖

12. Have you ever viewed yourself as a helpless victim to sexual temptation? According to Steve and Fred, what is a more honest assessment?

13. What is your reaction to the authors' definition of sexual purity? How would you rewrite it for single men?

EVERY SINGLE MAN'S WALK
(Your Guide to Personal Application)

📖 The simple truth? Impurity is a habit. It *lives* like a habit. When some hot-looking babe walks in, your eyes have the bad habit of bouncing toward her, sliding up and down....

The fact that impurity is merely a habit comes as a surprise to many men....

If impurity were genetic or some victimizing spell, you'd be helpless. But since impurity is a habit, it can be changed. You have hope, because if it *lives* like a habit, it can *die* like a habit. (We believe it can be done in six weeks.) 📖

📖 Don't misunderstand. We're not saying your habits have no relationship to your emotions or circumstances. Glen told us, "My sexual sin became much worse when I was under a deadline at work...or [when] I felt unloved and unappreciated. It seemed at those times that I was compelled to sin sexually and couldn't say no."

For Glen, job-related stress and lack of acceptance were not the *root* cause of his sexual impurity. The sexual impurity was simply one way he dealt with these emotions and circumstances. In short, he ran to impurity as an escape. But when he removed the sexual impurity, he began processing these things in other ways. 📖

14. Consider why the authors believe impurity and masturbation are habits. To what extent do you agree or disagree with their reasoning?

15. Think of some bad habits that you've killed in the past. Do you believe the impurity habit can die as well? What gives you hope?

16. Glen experienced an increased compulsion during times of stress, anger, or rejection. Can you relate? What could help you prepare for these times of particular vulnerability in the future?

17. a. What for you was the most meaningful concept or truth in this week's study?

b. How would you talk this over with God? Write your response here
as a prayer to Him.

c. What do you believe God wants you to do in response to this week's
study?

EVERY SINGLE MAN'S TALK
(More Topics and Questions for Group Discussion)

Key Highlights from the Book for Reading Aloud and Discussing

Because of rejection and lost love, men begin to seek for this lost love
in all the wrong places. In their search, where's the path of least resistance?
A pretend lover, a pornographic lover with a permanent smile. A lover
who never says no, one who never rejects. One who never abandons and is
always discreet. One who supports the man's ego in the midst of his self-
doubt.... This path is a chosen path, a path made available by the impure
eyes stoking the sexual fever, providing an unending pool of lovers from
which to draw.

While there may not be spiritual oppression involved in your battle,
there'll always be spiritual *opposition*. The enemy is constantly near your ear.

He doesn't want you to win this fight, and he knows the lies that so often break men's confidence and their will to win. Expect to hear lies and plenty of them.

📖 The first issue is accountability. For many men who are willing to fight for sexual purity, an important step is finding accountability support in a men's Bible study group, in a smaller group of one or two other men serving as accountability partners, or by going into counseling.

For an accountability partner, enlist a male friend, perhaps someone older and well respected in the church, to encourage you in the heat of battle. The men's ministry at your church can also help you find someone who can pray for you and ask you the tough questions. 📖

Discussion Questions

E. Which parts of chapter 10 in *Every Man's Battle* were most helpful or encouraging to you? Why?

F. What is your experience with seeking love in the wrong places? Do you agree this has been a choice? How does rejection or lost love tend to fuel this choice?

G. The authors say: "Expect to hear lies and plenty of them." Look at Satan's arguments listed under the heading Purity Always Brings Spiritual Opposition. Which of these arguments do you think are the most powerful and dangerous? Which of the truth responses are most encouraging to you?

H. Have someone read aloud the third quote above, dealing with accountability. Then go back to the conversation in the book between Ron and Nathan. As appropriate, talk together about how these kinds of relationships could work among some of the men in your group. Do any of the men want to set up an accountability relationship at this time?

1. Imagine what victory on the sexual battlefield would look like for you. How would you treat girlfriends and other women? How would you respond to visual temptation? What would your relationship with God be like? Now how are you going to get there?

victory with your eyes

Why must "bouncing the eyes" be immediate? After all, you might argue, a glance isn't the same as lusting. If we define "lusting" as staring open-mouthed until drool pools at your feet, then a glance isn't the same as lusting. But if we define lusting as any look that creates that little chemical high, that little pop, then we have something a bit more difficult to measure. This chemical high happens more quickly than you realize. In our experience, drawing the line at "immediate" is clean and easy for the mind and eyes to understand.

—adapted from chapter 11 in *Every Man's Battle*

EVERY SINGLE MAN'S BATTLE

(Steps Along the Path to Sexual Integrity)

Bouncing the eyes works.

You know what we're talking about—looking away when something sensual enters your field of vision. Bouncing the eyes breaks the addictive chemical cycle, and it's the key to breaking out of prison, no question. What many guys forget, however, is that outside the cell door is a long corridor with another heavy steel door waiting at the other end. To get out of the prison completely, you have to be *conformed* to act like Jesus (by bouncing the eyes) and—to get through the second door—you have to be *transformed* by the Word to think like Jesus. The following verse explains this well: "Do not be conformed to this world (this age), [fashioned after and adapted to its external, superficial customs], but be transformed (changed) by the [entire] renewal of your mind [by its new ideals and its new attitude]" (Romans 12:2, AMP).

Conforming is an act of the will regarding the choices you make in life, and that's what you're choosing when you bounce the eyes and starve the mind. But *transformation* goes well beyond your choices, because it reforms your will and your mind-set at the core.

Now some believe that temptation will always be there, like a parrot sitting on your shoulder, chirping away. They cite Paul's struggles with temptation and doing things he didn't want to do. Fair enough. We agree that Satan will never stop firing his grenades of temptation.

But is it really true that the power of Satan's temptations will always stay the same? Do you ever get to a point where fewer temptations are fired your way or at least the right choices are automatic?

Many would say no, but I (Fred) have seen Christ's beauty and majesty in my life. In light of that, I just can't think this way, and I don't think Paul meant for you to think that way either.

What I've found is that God is stronger in ways that we can never imagine, and He wants us strong as well. He wants us to see the way of escape, which He alluded to in this scripture: "When you are tempted, he will also provide a way out so that you can stand up under it" (1 Corinthians 10:13).

He wants you to be transformed into the same image of Christ from glory to glory (see 2 Corinthians 3:18) so that you can do even greater exploits (see John 14:12). If this is so, how can you say that the power of temptation never weakens or dies? If you do, that means you're saying that your tolerance level for temptation never changes—ever.

Come now! Do you actually think that Jesus struggled with this stuff throughout His adult life on earth? Does it make sense that the Lord, who sanctified Himself on our behalf, would leave us to struggle like this? No way, as this scripture confirms: "For their sake *and* on their behalf I sanctify (dedicate, consecrate) Myself, that they also may be sanctified (dedicated, consecrated, made holy) in the Truth" (John 17:19, AMP).

I've lived freedom, and I'm living it, just as Scripture promises. Sure, Satan would love to nail me, just as he'd love to nail you. He's fired his rocket-propelled grenades at me from time to time, but they've exploded harmlessly in the sands of the desert. He launched a shoulder-fired RPG the very night I signed the contract with WaterBrook to publish *Every Man's Battle*. I hadn't had a sensual dream about another woman in more than ten years, yet out of the blue, one happened. As the dream opened, I lay against a huge oak in the middle of a meadow with a nude, full-bodied woman sitting on my lap and gazing wantonly into my eyes. Quite an opening scene.

Without a trace of mental wrestling, I stood up, set her on the ground, and walked calmly away. Dream over.

Years ago I would have taken my fill of love with that gorgeous woman, but not this time around. Satan hit me at a high moment, thinking I had let my guard down. He wanted me to fall—by that I mean to lust after another woman in a dream—on the very day I signed the *Every Man's Battle* contract. That way he'd get me to question my fitness to be a spokesman for the principles of male sexual purity. Some say that the power of Satan's temptations never wane until we die, but I say that my dream proves that God's victory has sapped the power of Satan's temptations in my life.

Once He can trust you, God will give you a place of service fit for trustworthy men. God *wants* to freely bless you, and once He knows you've allowed His work to be completed in you, He also knows you're ready to fight on any battlefield.

If you're wondering what life is like on the other side of purity, here it is: "We, who with unveiled faces all reflect the Lord's glory, are being transformed into his likeness with ever-increasing glory, which comes from the Lord, who is the Spirit" (2 Corinthians 3:18).

EVERY SINGLE MAN'S TRUTH
(Your Personal Journey into God's Word)

Read and meditate upon the following Bible passages that have to do with the marvelous visual aspects of God's creation. Let the Lord bless you as you remember: He gave you sight that you might enjoy all the beauty and wonder of this world. The ultimate goal, of course, is that your heart may be lifted up in praise of His awesome power and glory. Why let your eyes pursue less worthy goals?

> O LORD, our Lord,
>> how majestic is your name in all the earth!
> You have set your glory
>> above the heavens....
> When I consider your heavens,
>> the work of your fingers,
> the moon and the stars,
>> which you have set in place,
> what is man that you are mindful of him,
>> the son of man that you care for him? (Psalm 8:1,3-4)

> The heavens declare the glory of God;
>> the skies proclaim the work of his hands.
> Day after day they pour forth speech;
>> night after night they display knowledge.
> There is no speech or language
>> where their voice is not heard. (Psalm 19:1-3)

> My eyes are ever on the LORD,
>> for only he will release my feet from the snare. (Psalm 25:15)

1. Consider the majesty of God conveyed by the heavens. When have you experienced this awesomeness in a night sky? Give thanks!

2. How can the creation "display knowledge"? What have you seen of God in nature?

3. If you've been using your eyes more for lust than for worship, what would you like to say to the Lord about that right now? Consider: what practical actions might help you to keep your eyes "ever on the LORD" this day?

☑ EVERY SINGLE MAN'S CHOICE

(Questions for Personal Reflection and Examination)

> 📖 A red-blooded American male can't watch a major sporting event without being assaulted by commercials showing a bunch of half-naked women cavorting on some beach with some beer-soaked yahoos. What's a man to do? 📖

📖 To attain sexual purity as we defined it, we must starve our eyes of the bowls of sexual gratification that come from outside…marriage. [You must] starve your eyes and eliminate "junk sex" from your life. 📖

4. Think about the red-blooded American male's dilemma in front of the television set. What is Fred's solution? Define "bouncing the eyes."

5. How many bowls of gratification do you think you receive from "junk sex" in a typical day? What will starving the eyes look like for you?

👟 EVERY SINGLE MAN'S WALK
(Your Guide to Personal Application)

📖 I [Fred] can't define the best defense for your weaknesses, but let me share mine so you'll get a feel for the process.…

Rule 1: When my hand reached for a magazine or insert, if I sensed in even the slightest way that my underlying motive was to see something sensual, I forfeited my right to pick up that magazine or insert. Forever.

To be honest, this didn't work well at first. 📖

📖 My body began to fight back in some interesting ways....

Whenever I was taken in by one of these tricks, I'd bark to myself in sharp rebuke, "You've made a covenant with your eyes! You can't do that anymore." In the first two weeks, I must have said it a million times, but the repeated confession of truth eventually worked a transformation in me. 📖

6. Look over Fred's list of My Greatest Enemies in chapter 11. What would be on your list of sources of sensual images? (Spend plenty of time coming up with an accurate list that doesn't overlook any important areas.)

7. Now spend plenty of time coming up with defense tactics in each identified area.

8. Fred says he can't define the actual defense methods that will work best for you. But what did you think of his own rules? What about rule number one? What rules are you considering for yourself?

9. Are you ready for your body and mind to fight back as Fred's did? What forms of inner rebellion will you likely need to prepare yourself for in this battle?

10. In quietness, review what you have written and learned in this week's study. If further thoughts or prayer requests come to your mind and heart, you may want to write them here.

◉◉ EVERY SINGLE MAN'S TALK
(Constructive Topics and Questions for Group Discussion)

Key Highlights from the Book for Reading Aloud and Discussing

📖 Imagine that your current level of sexual hunger requires ten bowls of sexual gratification per week. These bowls of gratification *should* be filled from your single legitimate vessel, the wife whom God provided for you. But because males soak up sexual gratification through the eyes, we can effortlessly fill our bowls from other sources. 📖

📖 "Wait a minute, Fred," you say. "Cutting down from ten bowls to eight bowls seems unfair. I'm being cheated, all because I'm obeying God!"

I guarantee you won't feel cheated. With your whole sexual being now focused upon your wife, sex with her will be so transformed that your satisfaction will explode off any known scale. Yes, even while consuming fewer bowls. It's a personal guarantee....

You can count on a sexual payoff from obedience. 📖

Discussion Questions

A. Which parts of chapters 11 and 12 in *Every Man's Battle* were most helpful or encouraging to you? Why?

B. What is your reaction to the bowls analogy? How helpful is it for you to view your sexual need this way? Why?

C. While a married man who starves his eyes drops from ten bowls to eight, an unmarried man who does the same drops to zero bowls. Does that feel like being cheated to you? Why or why not?

D. How might accepting zero bowls *now* enable you to get more enjoyment from your eight bowls *later,* assuming you get married at some point?

E. Are you willing to accept zero bowls, even if that is what you're going to get for the rest of your life because you never get married? If so, what makes you willing?

Note: If you're following a twelve-week track,
save the rest of this lesson for the following week.
If you're on the eight-week track, then keep going.

☑ EVERY SINGLE MAN'S CHOICE

(Questions for Personal Reflection and Examination)

📖 You'll need a good Bible verse to use as a sword and rallying point.

Just one? It may be useful to memorize several verses of Scripture about purity, as they work to eventually transform and wash the mind. But in the cold-turkey, day-to-day fight against impurity, having several memory verses might be as cumbersome as strapping on a hundred-pound backpack to engage in hand-to-hand combat. You aren't agile enough.

That's why we recommend a single "attack verse," and it better be quick. We suggest the opening line of Job 31:

I have made a covenant with my eyes. 📖

📖 Your shield—a protective verse that you can reflect on and draw strength from even when you aren't in the direct heat of battle—may be even more important than your sword, because it places temptation out of earshot.

We suggest selecting this verse as your shield: "Flee from sexual immorality.... You are not your own; you were bought at a price. Therefore honor God with your body" (1 Corinthians 6:18-20). 📖

11. Why do you need a sword and shield according to this chapter? What is their value in your pursuit of sexual purity?

12. What are the merits of Job 31:1 as a sword verse? As a challenge to this verse, what thoughts or arguments do you think Satan and his forces would be likely to use?

13. What are the merits of 1 Corinthians 6:18-20 as a shield passage? As a challenge to this passage, what thoughts or arguments do you think Satan and his forces would be likely to use?

14. What aspects of the authors' strategy for bouncing and starving the eyes make the most sense to you? What questions do you still have about these plans?

EVERY SINGLE MAN'S WALK
(Your Guide to Personal Application)

📖 Suddenly an old girlfriend pops into your mind. Note the great difference in perspective between the following two possible responses:

1. Should I daydream about my old girlfriend right now?

2. I don't even have the right to ask such a question, because I don't have the authority to make that decision.

The first response implies that you have the authority and the right to make that decision. The second implies that the question itself is moot. 📖

📖 In the long term, do you still have to monitor your eyes? Yes, because the natural bent of your eyes is to sin, and you'll return to bad habits if you're careless. But with only the slightest effort, good habits are permanent....

After a year or so—though it may take longer—nearly all major skirmishes will stop. Bouncing your eyes will become deeply entrenched. Your brain, now policing itself tightly, will rarely slip anymore, having given up long ago on its chances to return to the old days of pornographic pleasure highs. 📖

15. What verses will you select for your sword and for your shield? Why?

16. You do not have quite all of the restrictions that a married man has—you might still be looking at single women as potential mates (in a sexually pure way, of course). Nevertheless, what are some of the important questions in the realm of sexual temptation that you no longer have a right to ask yourself simply because you belong to Christ?

17. What kinds of short-term results and reactions do you expect in your pursuit of sexual purity? What kinds of long-term results and reactions do you expect in your pursuit of sexual purity?

18. In your own life, what do you believe are the most important factors that will ensure the success of this entire strategy for purity through your eyes?

19. a. What for you was the most meaningful concept or truth in this week's study?

b. How would you talk this over with God? Write your response here as a prayer to Him.

c. What do you believe God wants you to do in response to this week's study?

👥 EVERY SINGLE MAN'S TALK
(More Topics and Questions for Group Discussion)

Key Highlights from the Book for Reading Aloud and Discussing

📖 Once on an overnight hotel stay, I walked down the hallway to the ice machine. On top of the machine was a *Playboy* magazine. Believing I had a right to choose my behavior, I asked myself this question: Should I look at this *Playboy* or not?

The moment I asked that question, I opened myself to counsel. I began talking pros and cons to myself. But far worse, I opened myself to Satan's counsel. He wanted to be heard on this issue....

Therein lies the power of temptation. You may fear that temptation will be too strong for you in this battle, but temptations honestly have no power at all without our own arrogant questions. 📖

📖 Looking back at the details of our plan, even we will admit that it all sounds slightly crazy. Defenses, brain tricks, bouncing your eyes, forfeiting rights. Man! We wonder if even Job would be a bit startled.

On the other hand, maybe we should expect a sound plan to look this way. Consider all the men who are called to purity, yet so few seem to know how to do it. 📖

Discussion Questions

F. Which parts of chapter 13 in *Every Man's Battle* were most helpful or encouraging to you? Why?

G. Have you ever been there at the ice machine with Fred? What did you do in a similar situation?

H. According to Fred, what is the problem with getting into a conversation with ourselves about how we should respond to a particular temptation?

I. Fred and Steve admit that their plan for purity may seem slightly crazy. Have you had that reaction during this course of study? Talk about it.

J. What kinds of adaptations does their advice need when applied to single men, in your opinion? What one or more points that they make do you want to be absolutely sure you carry away with you?

victory with your mind

This week's reading assignment:

chapters 14–16 in *Every Man's Battle*

The great news is that the defense perimeter of the eyes works with *you to build the perimeter of the mind. The mind needs an object for its lust, so when the eyes view sexual images, the mind has plenty to dance with. Without those images, the mind has an empty dance card. By starving the eyes, you starve the mind as well.*

—from chapter 14 in *Every Man's Battle*

EVERY SINGLE MAN'S BATTLE
(Steps Along the Path to Sexual Integrity)

I (Fred) slumped into the aisle seat on my flight to Dallas, where I would teach at a weekend men's retreat on sexual purity. As I rested my elbow on the armrest and lay my head on my hand, my eyes focused aimlessly as my fellow passengers filtered by. I was exhausted, and I hoped my seatmate would arrive quickly so that I could stand up one last time and then plop down to grab forty winks.

Presently, a young woman caught my eye with a faint smile and a nod toward her seat, which was next to mine. I stood up politely to let her squeeze in, and then I settled down to buckle in. About ten minutes after takeoff, I absent-mindedly glanced out the window at the billowing clouds. As I did, I noticed this young woman had already laid her head back to sleep, and her low-cut top was offering a feast for my eyes. My eyes were free to roam.

Was I tempted? Nah. I simply turned the other way. At this point in my life, a lingering peek down a woman's blouse wasn't going to happen. Regarding the pretty young woman sitting next to me, everything had already been settled in my mind years ago. Transformation is transformation.

But as I fell asleep, I pondered what could have happened at one time. My eyes could have roamed all over her, using her voluptuous body for my selfish pleasure without her consent. *No, it would've been worse than that,* I mused. *I'd have been using her without her knowledge!*

Then suddenly it hit me. Peeking down her shirt as she slept beside me would really be no different than, say, watching her through her window with a telescope as she undressed some evening. Using her here on the plane would have been just as premeditated, just as deceptive, and every bit as creepy as that.

I shivered at the thought. *Man, I never thought of it quite like that before—and to think I used to lust like that all the time!*

Some may wonder about my choice to do the right thing in the airplane, *So what? She wouldn't have known if you were looking or not!* That's irrelevant. I would have been using her for a sexual pop without her consent. That's just plain degrading for any of us.

Besides, the fact of the matter is that I'm not entitled to use someone else's girl in that way, so end of discussion. To do so would be old-fashioned lusting, and Jesus said that lusting is the same as doing: "You have heard that it was said, 'Do not commit adultery.' But I tell you that anyone who looks at a woman lustfully has already committed adultery with her in his heart" (Matthew 5:27-28).

Recently our senior-high youth pastor was fired for sexual misconduct with a vulnerable seventeen-year-old girl from our church. His dismissal barely raised an eyebrow with me because I'd seen the red flags flying for months.

The day after the firing, though, I was shattered by an incredible, indelible sight, something my heart begs to never see again as long as I live. It happened when Randy, my dearest old friend, stumbled shakily into my office, his face contorted nearly beyond recognition. His skin was a jaundiced yellow, with rage and torment scrumming for turf upon his face. The two emotions were each grabbing and losing whole portions of his face, vaulting about so rapidly and randomly that I was frightened.

"Fred...how could he?" Randy murmured. "She was so vulnerable... She needed him... How could this happen?" He then burst into heart-wrenching sobs.

Much later, as the emotions were finally ebbing away, Randy told me something I'll never forget. "Fred, I have dozens of young women working for me, and do you know what I hear constantly from them? They tell me, 'Randy, I've never been around a man like you. I've never been able to trust a man in my life—my father, my brothers, my cousins—nobody. You're the only man I've ever felt safe to be around.'"

The tears came rolling again. "I can't tell you how much I cherish those words and that responsibility I carry. I fight with every fiber of my being to honor those girls who work for me. Many of them have been raped or molested at home. They *have* to be able to see God in me. So how could anyone violate that trust, especially a pastor? I *have* to be honorable with them!"

I couldn't help thinking of this verse: "Do everything...so that you may become blameless and pure, children of God without fault in a crooked and depraved generation, in which you shine like stars in the universe as you hold out the word of life" (Philippians 2:14-16). Randy shines in this present darkness.

Guys, let's catch God's vision and light it up. It's time to start honoring women with our eyes and our minds. They're entitled to nothing less, and we're entitled to nothing more.

📖 EVERY SINGLE MAN'S TRUTH

(Your Personal Journey into God's Word)

As you begin this week's study, read and meditate upon the Bible passages below that deal with appreciating God's grace, love, and power. Remember that you can choose to fill your mind with thoughts of God's goodness throughout your day. Think on these things!

> Answer me, O LORD, out of the goodness of your love;
> > in your great mercy turn to me.
> Do not hide your face from your servant;
> > answer me quickly, for I am in trouble.
> Come near and rescue me;
> > redeem me because of my foes.
> > > (Psalm 69:16-18)

Praise be to the God and Father of our Lord Jesus Christ, who has blessed us in the heavenly realms with every spiritual blessing in Christ. For he chose us in him before the creation of the world to be holy and blameless in his sight. In love he predestined us to be adopted as his sons through Jesus Christ, in accordance with his pleasure and will—to the praise of his glorious grace, which he has freely given us in the One he loves. In him we have redemption through his blood, the forgiveness of sins, in accordance with the riches of God's grace that he lavished on us with all wisdom and understanding. (Ephesians 1:3-8)

Brothers, whatever is true, whatever is noble, whatever is right, whatever is pure, whatever is lovely, whatever is admirable—if any-thing is excellent or praiseworthy—think about such things. (Philippians 4:8)

1. Have you ever prayed the kinds of words that we find in Psalm 69? Like David, do you have confidence in God's goodness, love, and mercy?

2. Meditate upon the blessings proclaimed in Ephesians 1:3-8. Make a list of the spiritual riches bestowed upon you as an adopted son of the heavenly Father. How will you live as His son today?

3. To what extent will your mind need transforming if you are to carry out the apostle's command in Philippians 4:8?

☑ EVERY SINGLE MAN'S CHOICE
(Questions for Personal Reflection and Examination)

📖 Your mind is orderly, and your worldview colors what comes through it. The mind will allow impure thoughts only if they "fit" the way you look at the world. As you set up the perimeter of defense for your mind, your brain's worldview will be transformed by a new matrix of allowed thoughts, or "allowables."…

This transformation of the mind takes some time as you wait for the old sexual pollution to be washed away. It's much like living near a creek that becomes polluted when a sewer main breaks upstream. After repair crews replace the cracked sewage pipe, it will still take some time for the water downstream to clear. 📖

📖 Have you "lurked at your neighbor's door"? It could mean stopping by in the late afternoon, visiting your friend's wife for coffee, enamored by her wisdom, care, and sensitivity. You felt sorry for her as you've commiserated together over her insensitive, brutish husband. You held her as she cried. You were lurking at your neighbor's door. 📖

4. Why is the mind more difficult to control than the eyes? How will your eyes work together with your mind in your pursuit of sexual purity?

5. What do the authors mean by "lurking at the door" and "mental lurking"? What is your own experience with this?

EVERY SINGLE MAN'S WALK
(Your Guide to Personal Application)

📖 According to Jesus, doing it mentally is the same as doing it physically. 📖

📖 Currently, your mind runs like a mustang. What's more, your mind "mates" where it wills with attractive, sensual women. They're everywhere. With a mustang mind, how do you stop the running and the mating? With a corral around your mind. 📖

6. How seriously do you take Jesus's words in Matthew 5:28?

7. How would you explain the authors' corral concept as it applies to sexual purity in your thought life? What does the corral represent? What does it accomplish?

8. How useful do you think this corral concept can be for you?

9. In quietness, review what you have written and learned in this week's study. If further thoughts or prayer requests come to your mind and heart, you may want to write them here.

EVERY SINGLE MAN'S TALK
(Constructive Topics and Questions for Group Discussion)

Key Highlights from the Book for Reading Aloud and Discussing

The defense perimeter of the mind is less like a wall and more like a customs area in an international airport. Customs departments are filters, preventing dangerous elements from entering a country. The U.S. Customs Service attempts to filter out drugs, Mediterranean fruit flies, terrorists, and other harmful agents.

Similarly, the defense perimeter of the mind *properly processes* attractive women into your "country," filtering out the alien seeds of attraction before the impure thoughts are even generated. This perimeter "stops the lurking."

Jack: "I knew that kiss would end my career at my church, but I couldn't help myself."

Discussion Questions

A. Which parts of chapter 14 in *Every Man's Battle* were most helpful or encouraging to you? Why?

B. How would you explain the process, as outlined in this chapter, by which the mind cleans away old sexual pollution? What encouragement does understanding this process give you?

C. What do the authors mean by a "mental customs station"? Describe this process in practical terms.

D. What do the authors mean by "starving the attractions"? What would it mean practically in your life?

E. How can starving the attractions help when you are interested in a single woman but she has said clearly that she is not interested in you?

F. Recall Fred's story of his high-school crush on Judy—and the disastrous prom date that ended it. Fred said: "My attractions to Judy died that night. The facts did them in!" Describe a time when you had an unreasonable crush on a woman—until the facts did it in.

Note: If you're following a twelve-week track,
save the rest of this lesson for the following week.
If you're on the eight-week track, then keep going.

☑ EVERY SINGLE MAN'S CHOICE
(Questions for Personal Reflection and Examination)

📖 Think about two types of women who will approach your corral:
- women you find attractive
- women who find you attractive

Both categories have similar defenses, each designed to starve the attractions until she trots off toward the horizon. 📖

10. What are the most important principles for having effective defenses against impure thoughts regarding women you find attractive?

11. What are the most important principles for having effective defenses against impure thoughts regarding women who find you attractive?

12. What is your level of temptation toward wives of your married friends or girlfriends and fiancées of your single friends? toward old girlfriends with whom you had an immoral relationship in the past? toward non-Christian single women? How can you apply the authors' suggestions to help you in these areas?

EVERY SINGLE MAN'S WALK
(Your Guide to Personal Application)

📖 *Always* play the dweeb. Players flirt… Learn to un-flirt. Players banter… Learn to un-banter. If a woman smiles with a knowing look, learn to smile with a slightly confused look, to un-smile. If she talks about things that are hip, talk about things that are un-hip to her.... She'll find you pleasant enough but rather bland and uninteresting. Perfect. 📖

📖 It's not that you don't trust your friend's wife; it's that you don't want to start anything. She should be like a sister to you, with no hint of attraction between you.

You'll always have *some* relationship with your friend's wife, but limit it to when your friend is around. This isn't always possible, but [some] simple rules can shield you from surprise attacks within the corral. 📖

13. Review the four shields from surprise attacks related to friends' wives. Consider the practicality of each suggestion for your own life.

14. What do the authors mean by "playing the dweeb"? With what categories of women should single men play the dweeb, and with what categories of women do they perhaps not need to play the dweeb? How effective do you think the tactic can be in your own life?

15. In your own life, what do you believe are the most important factors that will ensure the success of the authors' entire strategy for purity (that is, bouncing, starving, corralling, playing the dweeb, and so on)?

16. a. What for you was the most meaningful concept or truth in this week's study?

    b. How would you talk this over with God? Write your response here as a prayer to Him.

    c. What do you believe God wants you to do in response to this week's study?

🎭 EVERY SINGLE MAN'S TALK
(More Topics and Questions for Group Discussion)

Key Highlights from the Book for Reading Aloud and Discussing

📖 For those women who are already within your corral, the situation becomes rather complicated. These women won't drift back to the horizon. They're in your corral today and probably will be there tomorrow and the next day. This means you must eliminate these attractions in some other way. 📖

📖 In *The Final Quest,* Rick Joyner writes, "Spiritual maturity is always dictated by our willingness to sacrifice our own desires for the desires of others or for the interests of the kingdom."

Purifying your eyes and mind is more than a command—it's also a sacrifice. And as you make that sacrifice, as you lay down your desires, blessings will flow. Your spiritual life will experience new joy and power, and your marriage life will blossom as your relationship reaches new heights. 📖

Discussion Questions

G. Which parts of chapters 15 and 16 in *Every Man's Battle* were most helpful or encouraging to you? Why?

H. What tactics were presented for maintaining pure thoughts in regard to old girlfriends and ex-wives? How do these tactics apply to your situation as a single man? What is your opinion of their effectiveness?

I. What tactics were presented for maintaining pure thoughts in regard to the wives of your friends? Why is it important to think through this strategy? (Spend several minutes talking about the practical implications for your group.)

J. For single men, when is it okay to flirt and when is it not okay? How can single men pursue potential mates in a way that is above reproach?

victory in your heart

This week's reading assignment:

chapters 17–18 in *Every Man's Battle*

We know that relationships can be complicated, and everything is not cut and dried. It doesn't help that we men are ill-equipped to understand women and relationships—even when we think we understand and we think we are doing well.

Having said that, I want you to know that you are a warrior of the Lord God Almighty. The battle for purity lies before you, and victory is yours for the taking. God is with you, and make no mistake, together you stand as a formidable duo on the battlefield.

You can—and will—win this battle.

—from chapter 19 in *Every Man's Battle*

EVERY SINGLE MAN'S BATTLE
(Steps Along the Path to Sexual Integrity)

When I (Fred) was growing up in the hallways and locker rooms of life in America, sex seemed to be your ticket into manhood. But after lying in the arms of too many naked women, even I discovered that sex didn't admit me there after all. So if sex isn't the ticket, what *is* the Christian guy's rite of passage into manhood?

Jesus grew up here on earth, living until His early thirties. What was *His* rite of passage when He was coming of age? Do you remember how Jesus went with His parents to Jerusalem when He was twelve years old to the Feast of the Passover? Jesus, who was obviously thinking for Himself, got caught up in discussions with the religious scholars at the temple and stayed behind when his parents left for home. When his mother finally found him and asked what He was doing, Jesus responded respectfully, "Why were you searching for me?… Didn't you know I had to be in my Father's house?" (Luke 2:49).

Being about our Father's business is our rite of passage into manhood. That's where it's at—seeking and defending God's purposes for our lives. It's simply standing shoulder to shoulder with God in His desires and purposes for you and for your girlfriend (if you have one). If single Christian men were consumed by God's purposes, it would first be reflected in their personal purity and how honorably they treated women.

We've met very few men consumed by treating women with the highest respect, and fewer still are consumed by purity, but both attitudes are God's desire for you. For sure, we've painted a picture of personal purity for you in this workbook. But what is your Father's business when it comes to your treatment of that special person in your life when you are dating? We're talking about cherishing her for who she is in Christ.

When you cherish a wife in marriage, it means you will love her for who she is today—just as you love yourself. It means that she would have far more in marriage than she would have had she stayed a single woman. Cherishing a girlfriend isn't much different: you will love her for who she is today (just as Christ loves her), and you will leave her better off for having known you.

Let's say you're asking yourself, *How far can I go sexually with this woman?* It simply is not enough to ask, "Where are your boundaries, sweetheart?" Sure, this question will help you. If you intend to cherish her sacrificially, you certainly can't be charging over her sexual bounds, can you? Her answer to this question will give you the lay of her land.

But what if her sexual boundaries aren't as tight as her Father would like them to be? Say she gives you the high sign for a bit of sexual frolic when you're alone together. Does it still dishonor her if you go ahead? Yes, because it dishonors her Father. You must cherish both of them to discover purity in your relationship.

You must find the *boundaries* of purity, no question. But because so much spiritually is riding on all this for the both of you, it's even better to seek the *center* of purity in your relationships. For instance, kissing is not technically foreplay. I have kissed Mom, my sisters, and even my Aunt Nadine with no sexual overtones at all. Kissing may be fine for you and your girlfriend. We have no problem with that in general.

But when I look back, I'm not at all certain that some kinds of kissing were best for Brenda and me during our courtship. Our more passionate kissing ignited sensual infernos in my mind and made it harder for us to remain pure together, and it did little to strengthen our relationship or ensure the success of our pending marriage. All pain, no gain.

Marking out general boundaries, such as kissing the lips is okay but deep kissing is not okay, can be useful. But in my relationship with Brenda, splitting hairs on this issue missed the point entirely. Kissing Brenda passionately took my mind into dark, lustful corners where it had no business going.

And let's not forget this: maybe *you* can handle the kissing just fine. But what if it lights *her* fires, leaving her struggling to stay inbounds? Make a sacrificial stand for her purity and for God's purposes.

Finally, remember that the point of this workbook is not to hammer God's rules into you. Our ultimate point is to strengthen your intimacy with God. Is what you're doing with her resulting in a closer relationship with Him? Does it glorify Him? Are you satisfied with Him alone? Or must you have a taste of her body as well?

By now you know the right answers to these questions. So be a man and go out there and glorify God with His tender creatures.

📖 EVERY SINGLE MAN'S TRUTH
(Your Personal Journey into God's Word)

As you begin this final study, take some time to read and meditate upon the Bible passage below that has to do with the beauty of the bride. Keep in mind that, for centuries, the Song of Solomon has been viewed as an allegory of how Christ feels for His bride (all believers).

> How beautiful you are, my darling!
>> Oh, how beautiful!
>> Your eyes behind your veil are doves....
> Your lips are like a scarlet ribbon;
>> Your mouth is lovely....
> All beautiful you are, my darling;
>> there is no flaw in you....
> You have stolen my heart, my sister, my bride;
>> you have stolen my heart
> with one glance of your eyes....
> How delightful is your love, my sister, my bride!...
> Your head crowns you like Mount Carmel.
>> Your hair is like royal tapestry;
>> the king is held captive by its tresses.
> How beautiful you are and how pleasing,
>> O love, with your delights! (Song of Songs 4:1,3,7,9-10; 7:5-6)

1. Do you sense Jesus's desire for you as part of His bride? In return, does your heart yearn for Him like this?

2. If you are in a dating relationship, do you cherish your girlfriend with something like the same selfless love with which Christ cherishes you?

3. If you are divorced, did a failure on your part to cherish your wife contribute to the demise of your marriage?

4. If you are hoping to be married one day, are you planning to make a commitment to cherish your wife, not just when she pleases you, but even when you find things in her that disappoint you?

☑ EVERY SINGLE MAN'S CHOICE
(Questions for Personal Reflection and Examination)

📖 Our final word for you: If cherishing is anything, it's loving your [Friend? Girlfriend? Future wife?] for who she is *this day*, not some other day down the line. It's making allowances for all the surprises and inconsistencies that were hidden until life spun her in its new direction.

Your [Friend? Girlfriend? Future wife?] has a heart that still beats like a little lamb's heart, a heart that still skips through meadows of hope and desire, longing for love. It may be difficult to see. Maybe her father was an alcoholic or an abuser who didn't protect her. Maybe she isn't much of a Christian. Maybe she was promiscuous before meeting you.

Maybe so. But we know some other things are also true.

In trust to you, she *did* forsake her individual freedom, believing you would provide love and protection.

She's God's little ewe lamb regardless of the pain and sin she's been through, and *He* has entrusted her to you.

Can you see into her soul? Does your heart warm to the task? Is there anything more noble than making a solemn promise to cherish your one and only? 📖

5. Review the teaching in Ephesians 5:25-33. Although it is addressed to husbands, what guidance might it also give to men who are dating or engaged? What are the right attitudes and convictions as taught in this passage? What are the right standards and ideals? What are the right actions and habits?

6. What does it mean to you to cherish your girlfriend (assuming you are dating)? How does that differ from cherishing a wife?

7. Think back to your past relationships with women, whether ex-girlfriends or ex-wives. What "contractual" conditions did you try to hold those women to? Were you aware of doing this? What now needs to change in your approach to women?

EVERY SINGLE MAN'S WALK
(Your Guide to Personal Application)

In my office I keep an eight-by-ten, black-and-white photo of Brenda when she was one year old. Her little eyes sparkle and are filled with the hope and joy of life, her mischievous smile apparent even then; her glowing, chubby cheeks radiating joy and a carefree spirit. That face is so full of expectations and wonder. I brought that infant picture to my office because it reminds me that I need to honor that hope.

8. If you are dating someone seriously, do you have a picture of your girlfriend as a child? If so, what reminders does it give you when you look at it?

9. What boundaries have you and your girlfriend established for your relationship? In what ways are you seeking not just the boundaries but the *center* of purity together?

10. What can you do today to more faithfully honor your girlfriend? What can you do tomorrow?

11. In quietness, review what you have written and learned in this week's study. If further thoughts or prayer requests come to your mind and heart, you may want to write them here.

12. a. What for you was the most meaningful concept or truth in this week's study?

b. How would you talk this over with God? Write your response here as a prayer to Him.

c. What do you believe God wants you to do in response to this week's study?

⊘🕸 EVERY SINGLE MAN'S TALK
(Constructive Topics and Questions for Group Discussion)

Key Highlights from the Book for Reading Aloud and Discussing

📖 What does the standard of Christ's relationship to His church have to do with our sexual purity? In our hearts, we often have selfish attitudes and expectations regarding our wives. When these expectations aren't met, we become grumpy and frustrated. Our will to maintain our outer defense perimeters is eroded. 📖

📖 Uriah knew his place. He was satisfied to be part of God's purposes, to fill his role.

To be like Uriah, we must know our place and be content with it. 📖

📖 In our society, we have "sensitivity training" and "cross-cultural enrich-ment" classes. We believe if we can only teach people the "right" feelings, they'll act correctly. In the Bible, however, God tells us the opposite: We're to first act correctly, and then right feelings will follow.

If you don't feel like cherishing, cherish anyway. Your right feelings will arrive soon enough. 📖

Discussion Questions

A. Which parts of chapters 17 and 18 in *Every Man's Battle* were most helpful or encouraging to you? Why?

B. When have you been grumpy and frustrated when your expectations for women in your life haven't been met? Can you share about a recent example? How do you typically retaliate for unmet expectations?

C. Under the heading How Cherishing Feels in chapter 17, look at the authors' paraphrases from the Song of Solomon. How would you analyze the feelings conveyed in these passages? How helpful are these passages as tools for understanding your proper emotional involvement with your girlfriend and (potentially) your future wife?

D. Look at the quotation above about Uriah and then review the story of David, Bathsheba, Uriah, and Nathan (from 2 Samuel 11–12) as summarized by the authors. This is probably a story you've read before. As you consider it again, what stands out to you now that you've carefully studied sexual purity and made a commitment to pursue it? What are the most important lessons this story has for Christian men today, whether they are married or not?

E. Do you agree that we're to first act correctly and then right feelings will follow? Why or why not? What is your evidence?

F. Take a moment to reflect on what you've studied and discussed during the previous weeks. Ask each man to comment on one or more of these questions:

1. What can you thank God for as a result of this study?
2. What do you sense that God most wants you to understand at this time about this topic of male sexual purity?
3. In what specific ways do you believe He wants you now to more fully trust and obey Him?

Remember, even if you never have a date again and never marry, God cherishes you with all His heart and honors you for honoring His standards of sexual purity.

don't keep it to yourself

If you've just completed the *Every Single Man's Battle* workbook on your own and you found it to be a helpful and valuable experience, we encourage you to consider gathering a group of other men and helping lead them through this workbook together.

You'll find more information about starting such a group on page 2, under the section Questions You May Have About This Workbook.

_____

Steve can be reached by e-mail at sarterburn@newlife.com.

Fred can be reached by e-mail at fred@stoekergroup.com.

_____

the best-selling every man series—for men in hot pursuit of God's best in every area of life

Go beyond easy answers and glib treatments to discover powerful, practical guidance that makes a difference in men's lives—and in their relationships with God, the women in their lives, their friends, and the world.

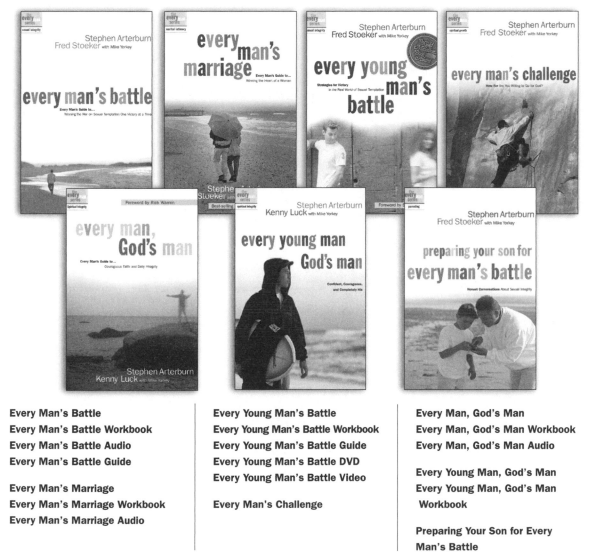

Every Man's Battle
Every Man's Battle Workbook
Every Man's Battle Audio
Every Man's Battle Guide

Every Man's Marriage
Every Man's Marriage Workbook
Every Man's Marriage Audio

Every Young Man's Battle
Every Young Man's Battle Workbook
Every Young Man's Battle Guide
Every Young Man's Battle DVD
Every Young Man's Battle Video

Every Man's Challenge

Every Man, God's Man
Every Man, God's Man Workbook
Every Man, God's Man Audio

Every Young Man, God's Man
Every Young Man, God's Man Workbook

Preparing Your Son for Every Man's Battle

For more information visit www.waterbrookpress.com. Available in bookstores everywhere.

 WATERBROOK PRESS

Helping women win the **battle** by **building** a strong **foundation** of **integrity**

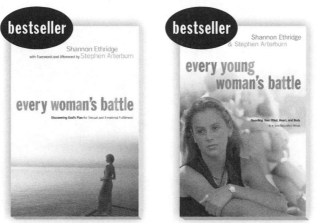

Companion workbooks are also available.

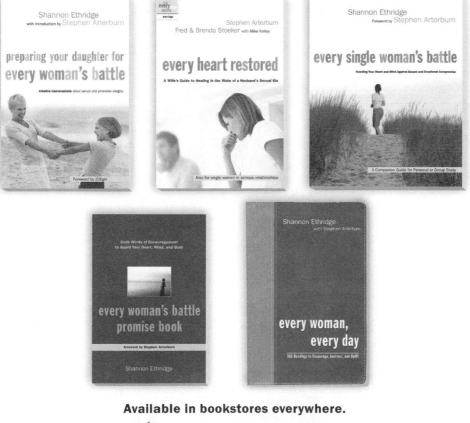

Available in bookstores everywhere.

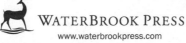
WATERBROOK PRESS
www.waterbrookpress.com